Ben Stacy Jerrik (Ed.)

Parent

Ben Stacy Jerrik (Ed.)

Parent

political, Childlessness, voluntary, pregnancy, infertility

Part Press

Imprint

Publisher:
Part Press is a trademark of
International Book Market Service Ltd., 17 Rue Meldrum, Beau Bassin, 1713-01 Mauritius
Email: info@bookmarketservice.com
Website: www.bookmarketservice.com

Published in 2012

Printed in: U.S.A., U.K., Germany. This book was not produced in Mauritius.

ISBN: 978-613-5-65691-6

Contents

Articles

References

Parent

A **parent** (from Latin: *parēns* = parent) is a caretaker of the offspring in their own species. In humans, a parent is of a child (where "child" refers to offspring, not necessarily age). Children can have one or more parents, but they must have two biological parents. *Biological parents* consist of the male who sired the child and the female who gave birth to the child. In all human societies, the biological mother and father are both responsible for raising their young. However, some parents may not be biologically related to their children. An adoptive parent is one who nurtures and raises the offspring of the biological parents but is not actually biologically related to the child. Children without adoptive parents can be raised by their grandparents or other family members.

A parent can also be elaborated as an ancestor removed one generation.

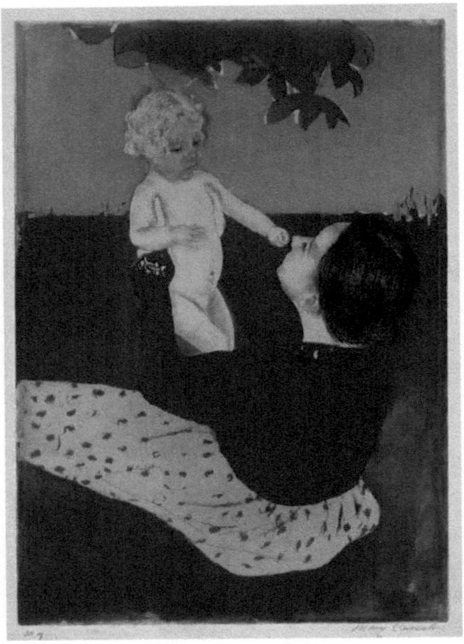

Under the Horse Chestnut Tree by Mary Cassatt, drypoint and aquatint print, 1898.

Biological and non-biological parentage

Like mothers, fathers may be categorized according to their biological, social or legal relationship with the child. Historically, the biological relationship paternity has been determinative of fatherhood. However, proof of paternity has been intrinsically problematic and so social rules often determined who would be regarded as a father e.g. the husband of the mother.

Biological parents and parental testing

The term *biological parent* refers to a parent who is the biological mother or father of an individual. While an individual's parents are often also their biological parents, it is seldom used unless there is an explicit difference between who acted as a parent for that individual and the person from whom they inherit half of their genes. For example, a person whose father has remarried may call his new wife their step-mother and continue to refer to their mother normally, though someone who has had little or no contact with their biological mother may address their foster parent as their mother, and their biological mother as such, or perhaps by her first name.

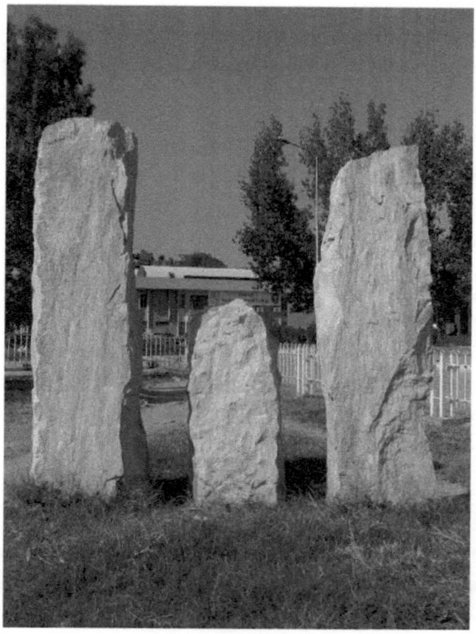

Monument to Parents and child

Parental problems

A paternity test is conducted to prove paternity, that is, whether a man is the biological father of another individual. This may be relevant in view of rights and duties of the father. Similarly, a maternity test can be carried out. This is less common, because at least during childbirth and pregnancy, except in the case of a pregnancy involving embryo transfer or egg donation, it is obvious who the mother is. However, it is used in a number of events such as legal battles where a person's maternity is challenged, where the mother is uncertain because she has not seen her child for an extended period of time, or where deceased persons need to be identified.

Although not constituting completely reliable evidence, several congenital traits such as attached earlobes, the widow's peak, or the cleft chin, may serve as tentative indicators of (non-) parenthood as they are readily observable and inherited via autosomal-dominant genes.

A more reliable way to ascertain parenthood is via DNA analysis (known as genetic fingerprinting of individuals, although older methods have included ABO blood group typing, analysis of various other proteins and enzymes, or using human leukocyte antigens. The current techniques for paternity testing are using polymerase chain reaction (PCR) and restriction fragment length polymorphism (RFLP). For the most part however, genetic fingerprinting has all but taken over all the other forms of testing.

Mother

A mother is a woman who has conceived, given birth to, or raised a child in the role of a parent.[1] Because of the complexity and differences of a mother's social, cultural, and religious definitions and roles, it is challenging to define a mother to suit a universally accepted definition. The male equivalent is a father.

Father

A father is defined as a male parent of any type of offspring.[2] The adjective "paternal" refers to father, parallel to "maternal" for mother. The verb "to father" means to procreate or to sire a child from which also derives the gerund "fathering".

Grandparent

Grandparents are the parents of a person's own parent, whether that be a father or a mother. Every sexually-reproducing creature who is not a genetic chimera has a maximum of four genetic grandparents, eight genetic great-grandparents, sixteen genetic great-great-grandparents, etc. Rarely, such as in the case of sibling or half-sibling incest, these numbers are lower.

Parent–offspring conflict

Parent–offspring conflict describes the evolutionary conflict arising from differences in optimal fitness of parents and their offspring. While parents tend to maximize the number of offspring, the offspring can increase their fitness by getting a greater share of parental investment often by competing with their siblings. The theory was proposed by Robert Trivers in 1974 and extends the more general selfish gene theory and has been used to explain many observed biological phenomena.[3] For example, in some bird species, although parents often lay two eggs and attempt to raise two or more young, the strongest fledgling takes a greater share of the food brought by parents and will often kill the weaker sibling, an act known as siblicide.

David Haig has argued that human fetal genes would be selected to draw more resources from the mother than it would be optimal for the mother to give, a hypothesis that has received empirical support. The placenta, for example, secretes allocrine hormones that decrease the sensitivity of the mother to insulin and thus make a larger supply of blood sugar available to the fetus. The mother responds by increasing the level of insulin in her bloodstream, the placenta has insulin receptors that stimulate the production of insulin-degrading enzymes which counteract this effect.[4]

Optimal gender mix

While a child has a biological father and a biological mother, not every family is a traditional nuclear family. There are many variants, such as adoption, shared parenting, step-families, and LGBT parenting, over which there has been controversy.

The social science literature rejects the notion that there is an optimal gender mix of parents or that children and adolescents with same-sex parents suffer any developmental disadvantages compared with those with two opposite-sex parents.[5] [6] The professionals and the major associations now agree there is a well-established and accepted consensus in the field that there is no optimal gender combination of parents.[7] The family studies literature indicates that it is family processes (such as the quality of parenting and relationships within the family) that contribute to determining children's well-being and "outcomes," rather than family structures, per se, such as the number, gender, sexuality and co-habitation status of parents.[6]

See also

- Bateman's principle – the theory that females almost always invest more energy into producing offspring than males, and that therefore in most species females are a limiting resource over which the other sex will compete.
- Borderline parents
- Child abuse
- Cinderella effect
- Egg and sperm donation
- Infant
- Narcissistic parents
- Non-paternity event
- Parental abuse by children
- Parental investment
- Parenting
- Parents bullying teachers
- Paternal bond
- Paternity (law)
- Reciprocal socialization
- Surrogate mother
- Teachers bullying parents

References

[1] "Definition from" (http://www.allwords.com/word-mother.html). Allwords.com. 2007-09-14. . Retrieved 2011-11-04.
[2] "WordNet" (http://wordnet.princeton.edu/perl/webwn?s=father). . Retrieved 2007-12-14.
[3] Trivers, R.L. (1974). "Parent–offspring conflict." *American Zoologist*, 14, 249–264.
[4] Haig, D. (1993). "Genetic conflicts in human pregnancy." *Quarterly Review of Biology*, 68, 495–532.
[5] Michael Lamb, PhD: Affidavit – United States District Court for the District of Massachusetts (2009) (http://www.glad.org/uploads/docs/cases/2009-11-17-doma-aff-lamb.pdf#page=13)
[6] "Elizabeth Short, Damien W. Riggs, Amaryll Perlesz, Rhonda Brown, Graeme Kane: Lesbian, Gay, Bisexual and Transgender (LGBT) Parented Families – A Literature Review prepared for The Australian Psychological Society" (http://www.psychology.org.au/Assets/Files/LGBT-Families-Lit-Review.pdf#page=8). . Retrieved 2011-11-04.
[7] "In The Supreme Court of Iowa No. 07–1499" (http://data.lambdalegal.org/in-court/downloads/varnum_ia_20090403_supreme-court-decision.pdf#page=10). . Retrieved 2011-11-04.

External links

- National Educational Network, Inc. (NENI) (http://www.neni.us) – free online resources for parent education, curriculum. They also have a parent blog with information about child care, afterschool, trends in education, tutoring, college, grants, etc.
- "Parents". *Catholic Encyclopedia*. New York: Robert Appleton Company. 1913. – A Roman Catholic view of the position of parents.

Offspring

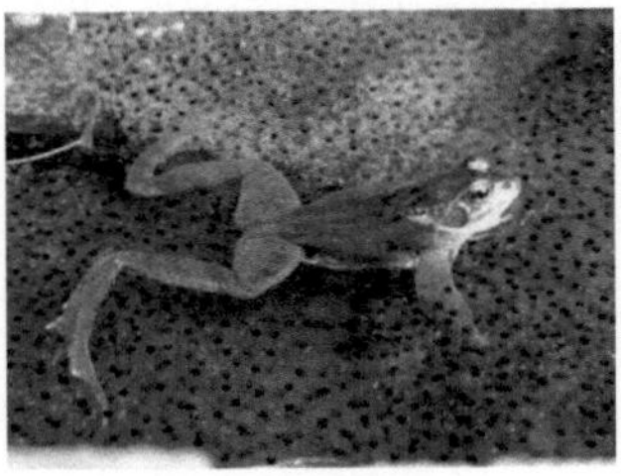
A frog in frogspawn.

In biology, **offspring** is the product of reproduction, of a new organism produced by one or more parents.

Collective offspring may be known as a **brood** or **progeny** in a more general way. This can refer to a set of simultaneous offspring, such as the chicks hatched from one clutch of eggs, or to all the offspring, as with the honeybee.

Human offspring (descendants) are referred to as children (without reference to age, thus one can refer to a parent's "minor children" or "adult children" or "infant children" or "teenage children); male children are sons and female children are daughters. See kinship and descent. Offspring can occur after mating or after artificial insemination.

See also

- Bateman's principle
- Clutch size
- Donor offspring
- Infanticide (zoology)
- Litter
- Parental investment
- Parent-offspring conflict

Ancestor

This article is about the concept of ancestry. For the website of the same name, see Ancestry.com. For the Scott Sigler novel by the same name, see Ancestor.

An **ancestor** or **forebear** is a parent or (recursively) the parent of an ancestor (i.e., a grandparent, great-grandparent, great-great-grandparent, and so forth).

Two individuals have a genetic relationship if one is the ancestor of the other, or if they share a common ancestor. In evolutionary theory, species which share an evolutionary ancestor are said to be of common descent. However, this concept of ancestry does not apply to some bacteria and other organisms capable of horizontal gene transfer.

Assuming that all of an individual's ancestors are otherwise unrelated to each other, that individual has 2^n ancestors in the nth generation before him and a total of about 2^{g+1} ancestors in the g generations before him. In practice, however, it is clear that the vast majority of ancestors of humans (and indeed any other species) are multiply related (see Pedigree collapse). Consider $n = 40$: the human species is more than 40 generations old, yet the number 2^{40}, approximately 10^{12} or one trillion, dwarfs the number of humans that have ever lived.

Ignoring the possibility of other inter-relationships (even distant ones) among ancestors, an individual has a total of 2046 ancestors up to the 10th generation, 1024 of which are 10th generation ancestors. With the same assumption, any given person has over a billion 30th generation ancestors (who lived roughly 1000 years ago) and this theoretical number increases past the estimated total population of the world in around AD 1000. (All of these ancestors will have contributed to one's autosomal DNA is concerned: this excludes Y-chromosomal DNA and mitochondrial DNA.)

Some cultures confer reverence to ancestors, both living and dead; in contrast, some more youth-oriented cultural contexts display less veneration of elders. In other cultural contexts, some people seek providence from their deceased ancestors; this practice is sometimes known as *ancestor worship* or, more accurately, *ancestor veneration*.

See also

- Cousin
- Ethnicity
- Family
- Family relationship
- Genealogy
- Kinship
- Most recent common ancestor

External links

- Ancestry.com corporate site [1]

References

[1] http://corporate.ancestry.com/

Generation

Generation (from the Latin *generāre*, meaning "to beget"),[1] also known as procreation in biological sciences, is the act of producing offspring. In a more general sense, it can also refer to the act of creating something inanimate such as ideas, sound, electrical generation using technology or cryptographic code generation.

A generation can refer to stages of successive improvement in the development of a technology such as the internal combustion engine, or successive iterations of products with planned obsolescence, such as video game consoles or mobile phones.

In biology, the process by which populations of organisms pass on advantageous traits from generation to generation is known as evolution.

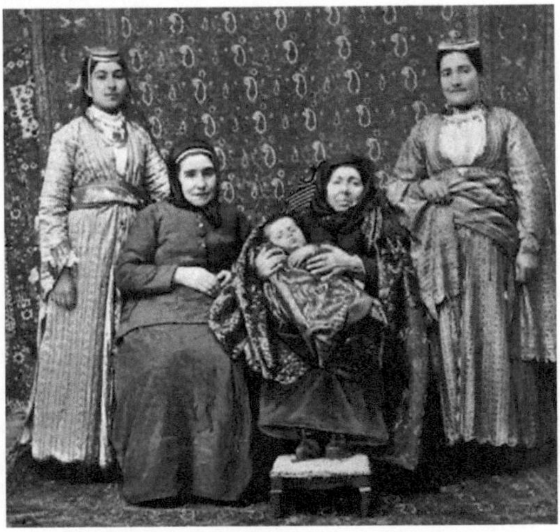

Five generations of one family: in the center, a child; on the far left, her mother; on the far right, the child's grandmother; second from the left, the child's great-grandmother; and second from the right, the child's great-great-grandmother.

Familial generation

Generational development can be both dependent upon cultural as well as circumstantial consequences. Society can influence the years between generations as can unforeseen situations. It is important to distinguish between familial and cultural generations. Some define a familial generation as the average time between a mother's first offspring and her daughter's first offspring. For much of human history the average generation length has been determined socially by the average age of women at first birth, about 16 years. This is due to the place it holds in the family unit economics of committing resources towards raising of children, and necessitating greater productivity from the parents, usually the male. With greater industrialisation and demand for cheap female labour, urbanisation, delayed first pregnancy, a greater uncertainty in relationship stability have all contributed to the increase of the generation length through the late-18th to the late-20th centuries. These changes can be attributed to both societal level factors, such as GDP and state policy, and related individual level variables, particularly a woman's educational attainment.[2] In developed nations the average familial generation length is in the high 20s and has even reached 30 years in some nations.[3] As of 2008, the average generation length in the United States was 25 years, up 3.6 years since 1970.[4] Germany saw the largest increase in generation length over that time period, from 24 years in 1970 to 30 years in 2008.[3] Conversely, generation length has changed little and remains in the low 20s in less developed nations.[3] <ref name="NCHS" generation are very important

Cultural generation

Cultural generations are cohorts of people who were born in the same date range and share similar cultural experience. The idea of a cultural generation, in the sense that it is used today gained currency in the 19th century. Prior to that the concept "generation" had generally referred to family relationships, not broader social groupings. In 1863, French lexicographer Emile Littré had defined a generation as, "all men living more or less at the same time."[5]

However, as the 19th century wore on, several trends promoted a new idea of generations, of a society divided into different categories of people based on age. These trends were all related to the process of modernisation, industrialisation, or westernisation, which had been changing the face of Europe since the mid-18th century. One was a change in mentality about time and social change. The increasing prevalence of enlightenment ideas encouraged the idea that society and life were changeable, and that civilization could progress. This encouraged the equation of youth with social renewal and change. Political rhetoric in the 19th century often focused on the renewing power of youth influenced by movements such as Young Italy, Young Germany, Sturm und Drang, the German Youth Movement, and other romantic movements. By the end of the 19th century European intellectuals were disposed toward thinking of the world in generational terms, and in terms of youth rebellion and emancipation.[5]

Two important contributing factors to the change in mentality were the change in the economic structure of society. Because of the rapid social and economic change, young men particularly were less beholden to their fathers and family authority than they had been. Greater social and economic mobility allowed them to flout their authority to a much greater extent than had traditionally been possible. Additionally, the skills and wisdom of fathers were often less valuable than they had been due to technological and social change.[5] During this time, the period of time between childhood and adulthood, usually spent at university or in military service, was also increased for many people entering white collar jobs. This category of people was very influential in spreading the ideas of youthful renewal.[5]

Another important factor was the break-down of traditional social and regional identifications. The spread of nationalism and many of the factors that created it (a national press, linguistic homogenisation, public education, suppression of local particularities) encouraged a broader sense of belonging, beyond local affiliations. People thought of themselves increasingly as part of a society, and this encouraged identification with groups beyond the local.[5]

Auguste Comte was the first philosopher to make a serious attempt to systematically study generations. In *Cours de philosophie positive* Comte suggested that social change is determined by generational change and in particular conflict between successive generations.[6] As the members of a given generation age, their "instinct of social conservation" becomes stronger, which inevitably and necessarily brings them into conflict with the "normal attribute of youth"— innovation. Other important theorists of the 19th century were John Stuart Mill and Wilhelm Dilthey.

Karl Mannheim was a seminal figure in the study of generations. He suggested that there had been a division into two primary schools of study of generations until that time: positivists, such as Comte who measured social change in fifteen to thirty year life spans, which he argued reduced history to "a chronological table." The other school, the "romantic-historical" was represented by Dilthey and Martin Heidegger. This school emphasised the individual qualitative experience at the expense of social context.

Mannheim emphasised that the rapidity of social change in youth was crucial to the formation of generations, and that not every generation would come to see itself as distinct. In periods of rapid social change a generation would be much more likely to develop a cohesive character. He also believed that a number of distinct sub-generations could exist.

Jose Ortega y Gasset was another influential generational theorist of the 20th century.

Since then, generations have been defined in many different ways, by different people. Generational claims can often overlap and conflict. Often generational identification has a strongly political implication or connotation.

List of generations

Western world

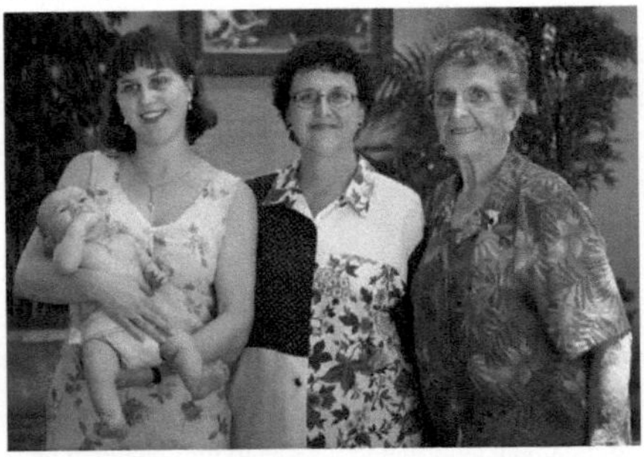

This photograph depicts four generations of one family: an infant, her mother, her maternal grandmother, and one of her maternal great-grandmothers.

- The Lost Generation, primarily known as the *Generation of 1914* in Europe,[7] is a term originating with Gertrude Stein to describe those who fought in World War I. The members of the lost generation were typically born between 1883 to 1900.
- The Greatest Generation, also known as the *G.I. Generation*, is the generation that includes the veterans who fought in World War II. They were born from around 1901 through 1924, coming of age during the Great Depression. Journalist Tom Brokaw dubbed this the Greatest Generation in a book of the same name.[8]
- The Silent Generation born 1925 through 1945, is the generation that includes those who were too young to join the service during World War II. Many had fathers who served in World War I. Generally recognized as the children of the Great Depression, this event during their formative years had a profound impact on them.
- The Baby Boom Generation is the generation that was born following World War II, from 1946 up to 1964, a time that was marked by an increase in birth rates.[9] The baby boom has been described variously as a "shockwave"[10] and as "the pig in the python."[11] By the sheer force of its numbers, the boomers were a demographic bulge which remodeled society as it passed through it. In general, baby boomers are associated with a rejection or redefinition of traditional values; however, many commentators have disputed the extent of that rejection, noting the widespread continuity of values with older and younger generations. In Europe and North America boomers are widely associated with privilege, as many grew up in a time of affluence.[10] One of the features of Boomers was that they tended to think of themselves as a special generation, very different from those that had come before them. In the 1960s, as the relatively large numbers of young people became teenagers and young adults, they, and those around them, created a very specific rhetoric around their cohort, and the change they were bringing about.[12]
- Generation X (also known as the 13th Generation and the Baby Busters)[13] is the generation generally defined as those born after the baby boom ended.[14] The term generally includes people born during all or part of the 1960s: According to Strauss-Howe generational theory, 1961 is the starting point, though other sources, including the U.S. Census Bureau, consider it to have started in the mid-1960s.[15] [16] It ends in late 1970s to early 1980s, usually not later than 1981[17] [18] [19] [20] or 1982.[21] [22] [14] [23] The term has also been used in different times and places for a number of different subcultures or countercultures since the 1950s.[24]
- Generation Y, the Millennial Generation (or Millennials),[22] [25] Generation Next,[26] Net Generation,[27] Echo Boomers,[28] describes the generation following Generation X. As there are no precise dates for when the Millennial generation starts and ends, commentators have used birth dates ranging somewhere from the mid-1970s[29] [30] [31] [32] [33] to the early 2000s (decade).[34] [35] [36] [37] [38] [39] [40] [41] Experts differ on the start date of Generation Y. William Strauss and Neil Howe use the start year as 1982, and end years around the turn of

the millennium,[42] [43] while others use start years that are earlier or later than 1982, and end years in the mid-1990s.[34] [44] [45] [46] [47] [48] [49] [50] [51] [52] [53] [54] [55] One segment of this age-group has often been called the “eighties babies” generation, in reference to the fact that they were born between January 1, 1980 and December 31, 1989.[56] [57] [58]

- Generation Z, also known as Generation I, or Internet Generation, and Generation Text,[59] and the "Digital Natives" by Marc Prensky and is the following generation.[60] The earliest birth is generally dated in the early 1990s.[61]
- Generation AO, the Always-On Generation (or Gen AO),[62] [63] [64] was first used by Elon University professor Janna Quitney Anderson in 2012 to describe people born between the early 2000s and the 2020s whose lives have been influenced since their early childhood by connectivity afforded by easy access to people and the world's knowledge through the Internet.[62] A survey of 1,000 experts she and Lee Rainie conducted for the Pew Research Center Internet & American Life Project found that the generation brought up from childhood with a continuous connection to each other and to information will be nimble, quick-acting multitaskers who count on the Internet as their external brain; the experts also predicted Gen AO will exhibit a thirst for instant gratification and quick fixes, a loss of patience and a lack of deep-thinking ability.[65]

Eastern world

- In China, the Post-80s (Chinese: or) (born-after-1980 generation) (also sometimes called China's Generation Y) are those who were born between the year 1980 to 1989 in urban areas of Mainland China. These people are also called "Little Emperors" (or at least the first to be called so) because of the People's Republic of China's one-child policy. Growing up in modern China, China's Gen Y has been characterised by its optimism for the future, newfound excitement for consumerism and entrepreneurship and acceptance of its historic role in transforming modern China into an economic superpower. Other Chinese generations are also named in a similar fashion, with Post-90s (Chinese:) referring to modern teenagers and college students.
- In South Korea, generational cohorts are often defined around the democratization of the country, with various schemes suggested including names such as the "democratization generation", 386 generation[66] [67] (also called the "June 3, 1987 generation"), that witnessed the June uprising, the "April 19 generation" (that struggled against the Syngman Rhee regime in 1960), the "June 3 generation" (that struggled against the normalization treaty with Japan in 1964), the "1969 generation" (that struggled against the constitutional revision allowing three presidential terms), and the *shinsedae* ("new") generation.[67] [68] [69]
- In India, generations tend to follow a pattern similar to the broad western model, although there are still major differences, especially in the older generations.[70] According to one interpretation, Indian independence in 1947 marked a generational shift in India. People born in the 1930s and 1940s tended to be loyal to the new state and tended to adhere to "traditional" divisions of society. Indian "boomers", those born after independence and into the early 1960s, tended to link success to leaving India and were more suspicious of traditional societal institutions. Events such as the Indian Emergency made them more sceptical of government. Generation X saw an improvement in India's economy and they are more comfortable with diverse perspectives. Generation Y continues this pattern.
- (From section "Post-80s in Hong Kong" of Post-80s) Post-80s in Hong Kong and the after-eighty generation in mainland China are for the most part different.[71] The term Post-80s () came into use in Hong Kong between 2009 and 2010, particularly during the course of the opposition to the Guangzhou-Hong Kong Express Rail Link, during which a group of young activists came to the forefront of the Hong Kong political scene.[72] They are said to be "post-materialist" in outlook, and they are particularly vocal in issues such as urban development, culture and heritage, and political reform. Their campaigns include the fight for the preservation of Lee Tung Street, the Star Ferry Pier and the Queen's Pier, Choi Yuen Tsuen Village, real political reform (on June 23), and a citizen-oriented Kowloon West Art district. Their discourse mainly develops around themes such as anti-colonialism, sustainable development, and democracy.[73]

Other generations

The term *generation* is sometimes applied to a cultural movement, or more narrowly defined group than an entire demographic. Some examples include:

- The Beat Generation, a popular American cultural movement that most social scholars say laid the foundation of the pro-active American counterculture of the 1960s. It consisted of Americans born between the two world wars who came of age in the rise of the automobile era, and the surrounding accessibility they brought to the culturally diverse, yet geographically broad and separated nation. The Beat Generation is between the Silent Generation and the Baby Boomers.
- The Hip Hop Generation, another popular American cultural movement describing a musical and cultural phenomenon that from humble beginnings had an international impact. Coined by author Bakari Kitwana, it describes a generation of people, regardless of race, who came of age in post-segregation America. Kitwana establishes the years 1965-1984, which includes Generation X and Generation Y.
- The Stolen Generation, a contentious term for children of Australian Aboriginal and Torres Strait Islander descent who were allegedly removed from their families by the Australian Federal and State government agencies and church missions, under acts of their respective parliaments between approximately 1869 and 1969.
- The Generation of €700 is a term popularized by the Greek mass media and refers to educated Greek twixters of urban centers who generally fail to establish a career. Young adults are usually forced into underemployment in temporary and occasional jobs, unrelated to their educational background, and receive the minimum allowable base salary of €700. This generation evolved in circumstances leading to the Greek debt crisis and participated in the 2010–2011 Greek protests.[74]

See also

- Generationism
- Intergenerationality
- Generational accounting
- Intergenerational equity
- Strauss-Howe generational theory
- Generation Gap

References

[1] "Generate | Define Generate at Dictionary.com" (http://dictionary.reference.com/browse/generate). Dictionary.reference.com. 1995-06-15. . Retrieved 2010-10-10.

[2] Bedasso, Biniam Egu. (http://www.uneca.org/acgs/mdgs/Education_Empirical_report.pdf) Investing in education as a means and as an end: exploring the microfoundations of the MDGs. United Nations Economic Commission for Africa Research Report, March 2008, accessed April 15, 2011.

[3] Organisation for Economic Co-operation and Development (OECD) Social Policy Division (http://www.oecd.org/dataoecd/62/49/41919586.pdf) SF2.3: Mean age of mothers at first childbirth, accessed April 15, 2011.

[4] Mathews TJ, Hamilton BE. (http://www.cdc.gov/nchs/data/databriefs/db21.pdf) Delayed childbearing: More women are having their first child later in life. NCHS data brief, no 21. Hyattsville, MD: National Center for Health Statistics. 2009, accessed April 14, 2011.

[5] Wohl, Robert (1979). The generation of 1914 (http://books.google.com/?id=YLe3e3FDXQkC&lpg=PA1&dq=wohl 1914&pg=PA1#v=onepage&q=). Cambridge, Mass.: Harvard University Press. pp. 203–209. ISBN 978-0-674-34466-2. .

[6] "Hans Jaeger. Generations in History: Reflections on a Controversy. Translation of "Generationen in der Geschichte: Überlegungen zu einer umstrittenen Konzeption," originally published in Geschichte und Gesellschaft 3 (1977), 429-452. p 275." (http://www.history.ucsb.edu/faculty/marcuse/classes/201/articles/85JaegerGenInHistHISTTHEO.pdf) (PDF). . Retrieved 2010-10-10.

[7] Wohl, Robert (1979). The generation of 1914 (http://books.google.com/?id=YLe3e3FDXQkC&lpg=PA1&dq=wohl 1914&pg=PA1#v=onepage&q=). Cambridge, Mass.: Harvard University Press. ISBN 978-0-674-34466-2. .

[8] Hunt, Tristram (2004-06-06). "One last time they gather, the Greatest Generation" (http://www.guardian.co.uk/uk/2004/jun/06/secondworldwar). *The Observer* (London). . Retrieved 2009-08-24.

[9] U.S. Census Bureau (http://www.census.gov/population/www/pop-profile/natproj.html)

[10] Owram, Doug (1997). *Born at the Right Time*. Toronto: Univ Of Toronto Press. p. x. ISBN 0-8020-8086-3.

[11] Jones, Landon (1980). *Great Expectations: America and the Baby Boom Generation*. New York: Coward, McCann and Geoghegan.

[12] Owram, Doug (1997). *Born at the Right Time* (http://books.google.com/?id=pKdw6Y7_lksC&lpg=PP1&dq=Owram, Doug Born at the Right Time&pg=PR11#v=onepage&q=). Toronto: Univ Of Toronto Press. p. xi. ISBN 0-8020-8086-3. .

[13] http://www.coachingandmentoring.com/Articles/x's.html

[14] Shin, Annys. "Non-Toxic Tots" (http://www.washingtonpost.com/wp-dyn/content/article/2008/02/29/AR2008022903658_pf.html). *The Washington Post*. . Retrieved 2010-05-03.

[15] "Special Age Groups" (http://www.census.gov/population/www/socdemo/age/general-age.html). U.S. Census Bureau, Population Division. . Retrieved 2012-02-06.

[16] Zimmerman, Eilene (2011-09-24). "Working Relationships Across Generations" (http://www.nytimes.com/2011/09/25/jobs/25career.html). *New York Times*. . Retrieved 2011-11-22.

[17] http://www.krusekronicle.com/2005/12/generation_x_19.html

[18] http://www.volunteeringinamerica.gov/special/Generation-X-%28born-1965-1981%29

[19] http://boards.ign.com/teh_vestibule/b5296/199231067/r199277178/

[20] http://www.uta.fi/FAST/US7/REF/genguide.html

[21] Rosenburg, Matt (2009-03-01). "Names of Generations (per the [[Population Reference Bureau (http://geography.about.com/od/populationgeography/qt/generations.htm)])"]. About.com. . Retrieved 2011-06-04.

[22] Strauss, William & Howe, Neil. *Generations: The History of America's Future, 1584 to 2069*. Perennial, 1992 (Reprint). ISBN 0-688-11912-3 p. 324

[23] Carlson, Elwood (2008-06-30). *The Lucky Few: Between the Greatest Generation and the Baby Boom* (http://books.google.com/?id=zUJgaHde6YUC&lpg=PP1&pg=PT45#v=onepage&q&f=false). Springer. ISBN 978-1-4020-8540-6. .

[24] Ulrich, John (2003-11-05) "Introduction: A (Sub)cultural Genealogy" (http://books.google.com/books?id=v10ZUR_Ca3EC&lpg=PA3&pg=PA3#v=onepage&q&f=false). In Andrea L. Harris. *GenXegesis: essays on alternative youth*. pp. 3. ISBN 978-0-87972-862-5. .

[25] Shapira, Ian (2008-07-06). "What Comes Next After Generation X?" (http://www.washingtonpost.com/wp-dyn/content/article/2008/07/05/AR2008070501599.html). *Education* (The Washington Post): pp. C01. . Retrieved 2008-07-19.

[26] "The Online NewsHour: Generation Next" (http://www.pbs.org/newshour/generation-next/index-old.html). PBS. . Retrieved 2010-08-24.

[27] Cheese, Peter (2008-03-13). "Netting the Net Generation" (http://www.businessweek.com/managing/content/mar2008/ca20080313_241443.htm?campaign_id=rss_null). Businessweek.com. . Retrieved 2010-08-24.

[28] Armour, Stephanie (2008-11-06). "Generation Y: They've arrived at work with a new attitude" (http://www.usatoday.com/money/workplace/2005-11-06-gen-y_x.htm). USA Today. . Retrieved 2009-11-27.

[29] Stephanie F. Gardner (August 15, 2006). "Preparing for the Nexters". *American journal of pharmaceutical education* (American Journal of Pharmaceutical Education) **70** (4): 87. doi:10.5688/aj700487. PMC 1636975. PMID 17136206. "born between 1976 and 1994"

[30] "Gen Y Propels Need for Online Service Technologies & Talent" (http://findarticles.com/p/articles/mi_m0EIN/is_2008_August_19/ai_n28010685). *Business Wire*. 2008-08-19. . Retrieved 2010-10-27. "born between the years 1976 - 1990"

[31] French, Dana (2005-11-21). "Generation Y versus Baby Boomers" (http://www.furnituretoday.com/article/32227-Generation_Y_versus_Baby_Boomers.php). Furniture Today. . Retrieved 2009-11-27. "Born between 1976 and 1994, more than one-third of Gen Y is still under 18."

[32] Price, Sarah; Kass, Susanna (2006-06-18). "Generation Y turning away from religion" (http://www.theage.com.au/news/national/generation-y-turning-away-from-religion/2006/08/05/1154198378623.html). Melbourne: The Age. . Retrieved 2009-11-27. "born between 1976 and 1990"

[33] Marquardt, Katy (2008-09-04). "Troubled Finances of the Young and Restless - New Money" (http://www.usnews.com/blogs/new-money/2008/9/4/troubled-finances-of-the-young-and-restless.html). usnews.com. . Retrieved 2010-08-24. "born between 1976 and 1987"

[34] "Is Your Firm Ready for the Millennials? - Knowledge@Emory" (http://knowledge.emory.edu/article.cfm?articleid=950). Knowledge.emory.edu. 2006-03-08. . Retrieved 2010-08-24. "born between 1982 and 2002"

[35] Tovar, Molly (August/September 2007). "Getting it Right: Graduate Schools Respond to the Millenial Challenge" (http://www.cgsnet.org/portals/0/pdf/comm_2007_08.pdf). *Communicator* **40** (7): 1. . Retrieved 2008-08-29. "born between 1982 and1994"

[36] Neuborne, Ellen (1999-02-15). "Generation Y" (http://www.businessweek.com/1999/99_07/b3616001.htm). Business Week. . Retrieved 2009-05-17. "Born during a baby bulge that demographers locate between 1979 and 1994"

[37] Bush, Alan J.; Craig Martin, Alan Bush, VVictoria Bush (2004-05-12). "Sports Celebrity Influence on the Behavioral Intentions of Generation Y" (http://journals.cambridge.org/action/displayFulltext?type=1&fid=216393&jid=JAR&volumeId=44&issueId=01&aid=216391). *Journal of Advertising Research* **44** (1): 108–118. doi:10.1017/S0021849904040206. . Retrieved 2010-10-28. "those individuals born between 1977 and 1994"

[38] By Nadira A. Hira, Fortune writer-reporter (2007-05-15). "Attracting the twentysomething worker. CNNMoney.com. May 15, 2007" (http://money.cnn.com/magazines/fortune/fortune_archive/2007/05/28/100033934/). Money.cnn.com. . Retrieved 2010-08-24. "for our purposes, those born between 1977 and 1995"

[39] "Demographics / Population Trends" (http://www.alliancetrends.org/demographics-population.cfm?id=34). Alliancetrends.org. . Retrieved 2010-08-24.

[40] Davis, Glyn (2005-05-30). "Rise of the millennials" (http://www.theage.com.au/news/Education-News/Rise-of-the-millennials/2005/05/27/1117129892594.html). *The Age* (Melbourne). .

[41] "How Generational Theory Can Improve Teaching: Strategies for Working with the "Millennials"" (http://www.worcester.edu/Currents/Archives/Volume_1_Number_1/CurrentsV1N1WilsonP29.pdf) (PDF). *Currents in Teaching and Learning* **1** (1): 29–44. Fall 2008. . Retrieved 2009-05-16. "Born between 1982 and 2003"

[42] Howe, Neil; Strauss, William (September 2000). *Millennials Rising: The Next Generation*. New York: Vintage. pp. 3–120. ISBN 978-0-375-70719-3.

[43] http://www.lifecourse.com/assets/files/yes_we_can.pdf

[44] * Tovar, Molly (August/September 2007). "Getting it Right: Graduate Schools Respond to the Millenial Challenge" (http://www.cgsnet.org/portals/0/pdf/comm_2007_08.pdf). *Communicator* **40** (7): 1. . Retrieved 2008-08-29. "born between 1982 and1994"

- Neuborne, Ellen (1999-02-15). "Generation Y" (http://www.businessweek.com/1999/99_07/b3616001.htm). Business Week. . Retrieved 2009-05-17. "Born during a baby bulge that demographers locate between 1979 and 1994"
- Bush, Alan J.; Craig Martin, Alan Bush, VVictoria Bush (2004-05-12). "Sports Celebrity Influence on the Behavioral Intentions of Generation Y" (http://journals.cambridge.org/action/displayFulltext?type=1&fid=216393&jid=JAR&volumeId=44&issueId=01&aid=216391). *Journal of Advertising Research* **44** (1): 108–118. doi:10.1017/S0021849904040206. . Retrieved 2010-10-28. "those individuals born between 1977 and 1994"
- By Nadira A. Hira, Fortune writer-reporter (2007-05-15). "Attracting the twentysomething worker. CNNMoney.com. May 15, 2007" (http://money.cnn.com/magazines/fortune/fortune_archive/2007/05/28/100033934/). Money.cnn.com. . Retrieved 2010-08-24. "for our purposes, those born between 1977 and 1995"
- "Demographics / Population Trends" (http://www.alliancetrends.org/demographics-population.cfm?id=34). Alliancetrends.org. . Retrieved 2010-08-24.
- Davis, Glyn (2005-05-30). "Rise of the millennials" (http://www.theage.com.au/news/Education-News/Rise-of-the-millennials/2005/05/27/1117129892594.html). *The Age* (Melbourne). .
- "How Generational Theory Can Improve Teaching: Strategies for Working with the "Millennials"" (http://www.worcester.edu/Currents/Archives/Volume_1_Number_1/CurrentsV1N1WilsonP29.pdf) (PDF). *Currents in Teaching and Learning* **1** (1): 29–44. Fall 2008. . Retrieved 2009-05-16. "Born between 1982 and 2003"

[45] McCrindle, Mark (2005-07-18). "Superannuation and the Under 40's: Summary Report: Research Report on the Attitudes and Views of Generations X and Y on Superannuation" (www.aph.gov.au/house/committee/efpa/super/subs/sub002.pdf). *McCrindle Research*. "Generation X comprises those aged between 24 and 40...Generation Y 1982-2000..."

[46] Kershaw, Pam (2005). "Managing Generation X and Y" (http://www.kershaw.com.au/popup/editorial_05.html). *The Sydney Morning Herald* (Fairfax Media). . Retrieved 2010-12-18. "Mark McCrindle, director of McCrindle Research Pty Ltd which specialises in social and generational studies, says differences between generations in the workplace have never been greater...Generation Y: born 1982 onwards, aged 23 or younger."

[47] Shoebridge, Neil (2006-10-11). "Generation Y: Catch Them If You Can" (http://www.id.co.nz/138a1.page). *Australian Financial Review* (Fairfax Media). . Retrieved 2010-12-18. "The definitions of generation Y vary...others plumping for 1982 to 1995."

[48] "State of the News Print Media in Australia Report 2008" (http://www.presscouncil.org.au/snpma/snpma2008/ch08_2_snpma2008.html). Australian Press Council. 2008-12-22. . Retrieved 2010-12-18. "This comment is not meant to convey a negative in regard Generation X (1965–1981) and Generation Y (1982–2000)."

[49] "Generation X and Y: Who They Are and What They Want" (http://www.governance.com.au/board-matters/fx-view-article.cfm?loadref=2&article_id=EB2FC50B-8C97-4666-861D7BB0EEF306AF). *Board Matters Newsletter* **8** (3). 2008-11. . Retrieved 2010-12-18. "Generation Y 1982-2000"

[50] "Achievement for All Children: An Apple Canada Perspective" (http://www.bcssa.org/) (www.bcssa.org/topics/WhitePaper_Canada_CE.pdf). *Apple Canada*. Apple Inc.. 2004-04-19. . Retrieved 2010-12-19. "Generation Y, or the 'Millennials,' as they prefer to be called, are the children of the Boomers and early-wave members of Generation X. They account for almost 26% of Canada's population. Born between 1982 and 2000, this first generation of the new millennium populates classes in elementary, middle, and high schools, as well as colleges and universities."

[51] Crealock, Martha (2008-Jan.). "The Teachers Write – About Millennials" (www.usask.ca/gmcte/drupal/files/bridges_Jan08.pdf). *Bridges* **6** (2): 10–11. "This issue's topic is the Millennials. There has been a lot of talk about 'Millennials,' or "Generation Y": young people born between 1982 - 2000."

[52] "Generation Y: Challenging Employers to Provide Balance: Who are Generation Y and do employers and managers in the non-profit sector really need to fear them?" (http://www.bccf.ca/all/resources/generation-y-challenging-employers-provide-balance). *Family Connections* **12** (2). 2008-Summer. . Retrieved 2010-12-19. "Generation Y – also frequently known as the Echo Boomers, the Millenials, the Net Generation, or the Next Generation – are those people born between 1982 and 1997."

[53] "Millennials & The Digital Entertainment Age: A Sourcebook for Consumer Marketers" (http://www.millennialsconference.com/canada/). *The Millennials*. Toronto, Canada: Digital Media Wire. 2008-03-05. . "By the year 2010, Millennials, born between 1982 and 1993, will outnumber both Baby Boomers and Gen-Xers and will be the most significant consumer sector for the media & entertainment industries."

[54] "Destination Canada: Are We Doing Enough?" (http://www.linkbc.ca/torc/downs1/Destionationcanadav3.pdf). *Deloitte Tourism, Hospitality & Leisure Industry and Tourism Industry Association of Canada (TIAC)*: 1–16. 2009. . Retrieved 2011-03-28. "67% are members of Generations X (1961-81) and Y (1982-2001), or the 'contemporary generations'"

[55] Joel, Mitch (2010-10-14). "Social Media a Waste of Time? Not to Gen Y" (http://www.vancouversun.com/business/technology/Social+media+waste+time/3669581/story.html). *The Vancouver Sun* (Pacific Newspaper Group). . Retrieved 2010-12-19. "Contrast the news above with this blog post last week from MediaPost's Engage — Gen Y titled, Social Network Disconnect (Oct. 8), which looks at generation Y (those born between 1982 and 1993)."

[56] "The Millennial Manifesto: How 80's Babies Can Save the World. by Jermaine Spradley +" (http://www.huffingtonpost.com/jermaine-spradley/a-millennial-manifesto-jobs_b_956053.html). huffingtonpost.com. 2011-09-11. . Retrieved 2011-11-22.

[57] "Economic 'boom': '80s babies get set to flex spending power. by Richard Burnett" (http://articles.orlandosentinel.com/2007-05-26/news/ECHOSPEND26_1_echo-boomers-baby-boomers-visa-usa). orlandosentinal.com. 2007-05-26. . Retrieved 2011-11-22.

[58] "Pity the plight of the 80s babies. by ChrisGiles" (http://www.ft.com/intl/cms/s/0/b97ad1c2-30d8-11dc-9a81-0000779fd2ac.html#axzz1ePPzoUxz). financialtimes.com. 2007-07-13. . Retrieved 2011-11-22.

[59] http://www.buffalonews.com/topics/back-to-school/article522374.ece

- Leonard, Bill (January 2000). "After Generations X and Y Comes Generation I - Internet generation - Brief Article" (http://findarticles.com/p/articles/mi_m3495/is_1_45/ai_59283651/). *BNET (Orig. HR Magazine)*. . Retrieved 10 February 2010.
- "The Challenge and Promise of "Generation I"" (http://www.microsoft.com/presspass/features/1999/10-28geni.mspx) (Press release). Microsoft. 28 October 1999. . Retrieved 10 February 2010.
- Gardner, John William; Bryn Holmes (2006). *E-Learning: Concepts and Practice*. London: Sage Publications Ltd. pp. 61 (http://books.google.ca/books?id=XbbM9mj22KQC&pg=PA61). ISBN 1-4129-1111-7.
- Posnick-Goodwin, Sherry (February 2010). "Meet generation Z" (http://www.cta.org/Professional-Development/Publications/Educator-Feb-10/Meet-Generation-Z.aspx). *California Teachers Association*. . Retrieved 2010-06-15.
- Schmidt, Lucinda; Hawkins, Peter (2008-07-18). "Gen Z: digital natives" (http://www.essentialbaby.com.au/toddler/gen-z-digital-natives-20080716-3g5p.html?page=-1). *essentialbaby.com.au*. . Retrieved 2010-06-15.
- Mitchell, David (2008-08-16). "Generation Z-striking the balance" (http://www.ncbi.nlm.nih.gov/pubmed/18704218). *National Center for Biotechnology Information*. . Retrieved 2010-06-15.
- Schmidt, Lucinda; Hawkins, Peter (July 15, 2008). "Children of the tech revolution" (http://www.smh.com.au/news/parenting/children-of-the-tech-revolution/2008/07/15/1215887601694.html). Sydney Morning Herald. .
- Tapscott, Don (2008). *Grown Up Digital: How the Net Generation is Changing Your World*. McGraw-Hill. pp. 15–16. ISBN 978-0-07-150863-6.
- Walliker, Annalise (25 February 2008). "Generation Z comes of age" (http://www.news.com.au/heraldsun/story/0,21985,23269842-662,00.html). Herald Sun. . Retrieved 27 April 2009.

[62] Quitney Anderson, Janna (2012-02-29). "What is the likely future of Generation AO in 2020?" (http://www.elon.edu/e-web/predictions/expertsurveys/2012survey/default.xhtml). *education*. Imagining the Internet Center Elon University. .

[63] Gregory, Ted (2012-02-29). "Eternal discipline: The price of managed hyperconnectivity" (http://www.chicagotribune.com/news/local/ct-met-millennials-sidebar-20120229,0,902645.story). The Chicago Tribune. . Retrieved 2012-02-29.

[64] Netburn, Deborah (2012-02-29). "Pew study: Is the Internet ruining or improving today's youth?" (http://www.latimes.com/business/technology/la-fi-tn-pew-research-future-of-internet-survey-20120228,0,6379504.story). The Los Angeles Times. . Retrieved 2012-02-29.

[65] Anderson, Janna (2012-02-29). "Hyperconnected will benefit and suffer" (http://www.pewinternet.org/Reports/2012/Hyperconnected-lives.aspx). *research*. Pew Research Center's Internet & American Life Project. .

[66] "Fiasco of 386 Generation" (http://www.koreatimes.co.kr/www/news/special/2008/04/180_18529.html). Koreatimes.co.kr. . Retrieved 2010-10-10.

[67] "Shinsedae: Conservative Attitudes of a 'New Generation' in South Korea and the Impact on the Korean Presidential Election" (http://www.eastwestcenter.org/news-center/east-west-wire/shinsedae-conservative-attitudes-of-a-new-generation-in-south-korea-and-the-impact-on-the-korean-presidential-election/). Eastwestcenter.org. . Retrieved 2010-10-10.

[68] **(Korean)** http://www.koreaherald.co.kr/NEWKHSITE/data/html_dir/2009/08/26/200908260078.asp

[69] (http://www.ekoreajournal.net/upload/pdf/PDF4033M)

[70] "Generational Differences Between India and the U.S" (http://blogs.harvardbusiness.org/erickson/2009/02/global_generations_focus_on_in.html). Blogs.harvardbusiness.org. 2009-02-28. . Retrieved 2010-10-10.

[71] Post 80s rebels with a cause (http://www.thestandard.com.hk/news_detail.asp?we_cat=12&art_id=93121&sid=26708529&con_type=3&d_str=20100115&fc=4), The Standard, Coleen Lee, 15 Jan 2010, Accessed 20 Jun 2010

[72] Kwong wing-yuen (ed.), Zhan zai dan de yi bian, Xianggang bashihou, Hong Kong, UP Publications Limited, 2010, pp. 16-32.

[73] "From the Star Ferry Pier to the Express Rail : emancipate the city and the citizen - Analysis of Hong Kong's new civil society" Le mouvement civique urbain hongkongais Emanciper la ville et le citoyen (http://www.scribd.com/doc/34334722/Pierre-Martin-Du-Star-Ferry-a-l-Express-Rail-analyse-de-la-nouvelle-societe-civile-hongkongaise-From-the-Star-Ferry-Pier-to-the-Express-Rail-an) **(French)**

[74] http://www.dw-world.de/dw/article/0,,15117098,00.html

- William Strauss and Neil Howe (1991) *Generations: The History of America's Future, 1584-2069,* ISBN 0-688-11912-3

External links

- Generations and Population (http://members.optusnet.com.au/exponentialist/Generations_and_Population_Doublings.htm)
- Resources on the Generations (http://www.mccrindle.com.au/resources.htm)

Birth

Birth (**calving** in livestock and some other animals, **whelping** in carnivorous mammals) is the act or process of bearing or bringing forth offspring.[1] The offspring is brought forth from the mother. The time of human birth is defined as the time at which the fetus comes out of the mother's womb into the world. Different forms of birth are oviparity, vivipary and ovovivipary.

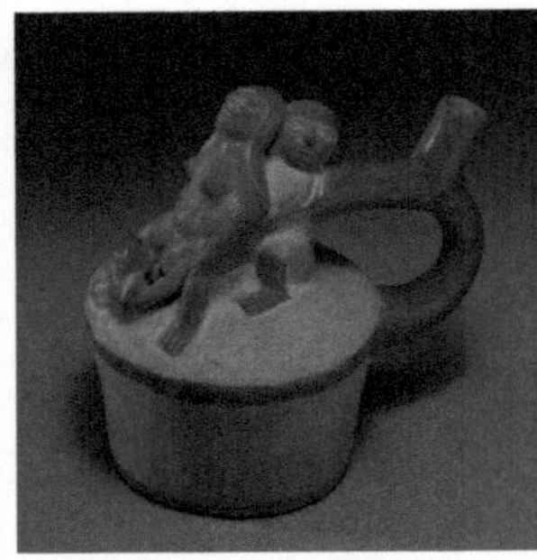

Moche ceramic vessel showing a woman giving birth. Larco Museum Collection. Lima-Peru

Medical meanings

- Afterbirth is the birth of the placenta following the birth of the infant.
- Birth canal is the term used for the vagina during birth, as it is the route through which the infant passes during a vaginal birth.
- Birth control methods are devices, medications or behavior patterns employed to reduce the probability of pregnancy.
- Birth doula is the term for a labor assistant that provides emotional support, physical comfort measures, and other assistance to expecting mothers, partners, families, and baby before, during, and after childbirth. A postpartum doula provides support after birth, and specializes in postpartum care for mother and infant, infant attachment, and other newborn care. The term "doula" stems from the Greek *doulos*, or "one who serves."
- Birth pangs are the pains felt by the mother during labor, resulting from contractions of the uterus and pressure on nerves and organs.
- Caesarean section or C-section is surgical birth through the wall of the abdomen.
- Childbirth is the process at the end of a human pregnancy that results in a baby being born.
- Lotus birth is the practice of leaving the umbilical cord uncut after birth so that the baby is left attached to its placenta until the cord naturally separates.
- Midwife is the term for a health care provider that provides at home health care for expecting mothers, delivers baby during birth, and provides postpartum care.

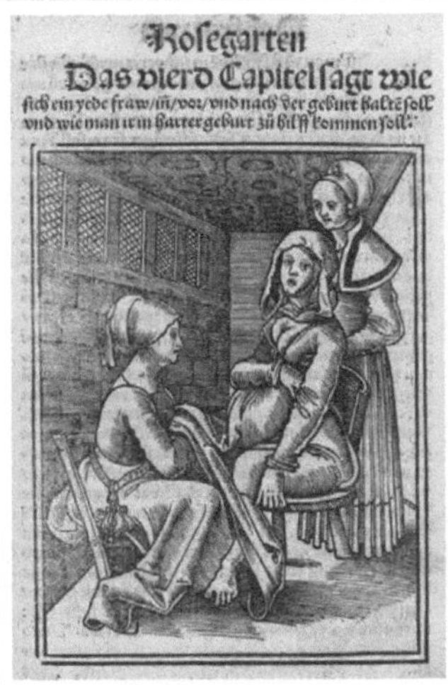

A woman giving birth on a birth chair, circa 1515

- Multiple birth is the birth of two (twins), three (triplets), four (quadruplets), etc., babies resulting from a single pregnancy.
- Natural childbirth is the technique of minimizing medical intervention, particularly anaesthetics, during childbirth.

- Placenta is the organ in most female mammals, formed in her lining of the uterus by the union of the uterine mucus membrane with the membranes of the fetus, that provides for the nourishment of the fetus and the elimination of its waste products.[2]
- Unassisted childbirth (UC) is birth without the aid of medical or professional birth attendants. Also known as freebirth

Complications

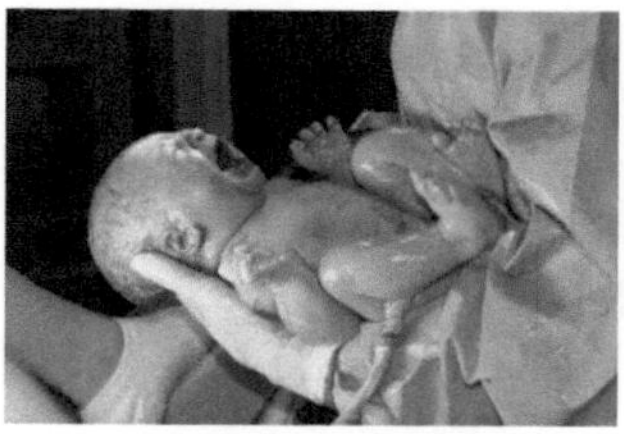
Newborn after typical hospital birth

- Birth defect is a physical or mental abnormality present at the time of birth.
- Birth trauma is a theory in Pre & Perinatal psychology and natural medicine that the baby experiences extreme pain during the birthing process and that this pain influences the child later in life.
- Complications may cause a miscarriage or spontaneous abortion to occur.[3]
- Infertility treatments are devices, medications, or behavior patterns to increase the probability of pregnancy.
- Musculoskeletal disorders. Pregnancy related Pelvic Girdle Pain is a significant musculoskeletal disorder that begins in pregnancy and for some women last for years.
- Premature birth is the birth of an infant before the full term of pregnancy.
- Stillbirth is the birth of a dead fetus or infant.
- VBAC is a Vaginal Birth after a Caesarean Birth.

Legal meanings

- Birth certificate is a legal document describing details of a person's birth.
- Birthday is a day to celebrate that the person has lived a certain number of years. It is an annual event based either on the anniversary of a person's date of birth, or on astrological birthtime calculations.
- A nuclear family comprising the father, mother, brother or sister, is an institution where the members are related by birth.
- In some countries a person is considered of illegitimate birth if the child is born of parents not legally married to one another.

Spiritual meanings

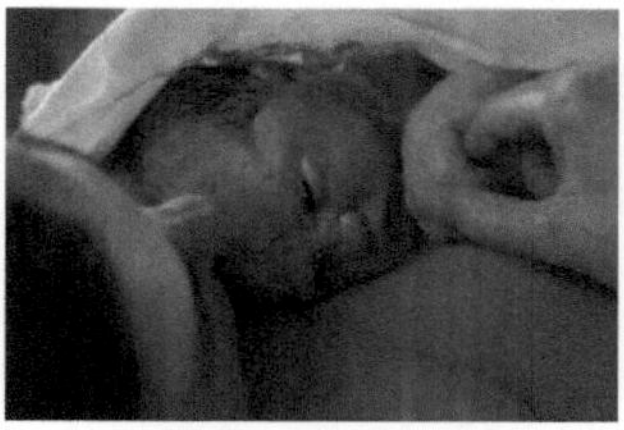
Mother and child union, immediately after birth

- Astrology is based upon the belief that an individual's life is influenced by the geocentric positions of the Sun, Moon, and planets in the sky or below the horizon at the moment of birth; a natal chart is calculated using the exact time, date, and place of birth to try to interpret these cyclical influences on a person's life.
- Born again, a term used primarily in Protestant Christianity, is associated with salvation, conversion, and spiritual rebirth.
- Rebirth is a belief that a person is born again after their death based on the karma of their previous births.
- Virgin birth of Jesus is the Christian doctrine that asserts that Jesus Christ was born to a virgin, and thus that his conception was carried out without an earthly father.

See also

- Childbirth
- Death
- Fertilization
- Home birth
- List of oldest birth mothers
- List of youngest birth mothers
- Pregnancy
- Prenatal nutrition and birth weight
- Storks
- Whelping

References

[1] Birth (http://dictionary.reference.com/browse/birth), dictionary.com, Retrieved on June 10, 2010.

[2] Dictionary.reference.com (http://dictionary.reference.com/search?q=Placenta)

[3] Hurwitz, J. and J. Leis (1972). "Directing influence of DNA in the reaction". *RNA-dependent DNA polymerase activity of RNA tumor viruses*. pp. 116–129.

Interpersonal_relationship

An **interpersonal relationship** is an association between two or more people that may range from fleeting to enduring. This association may be based on inference, love, solidarity, regular business interactions, or some other type of social commitment. Interpersonal relationships are formed in the context of social, cultural and other influences. The context can vary from family or kinship relations, friendship, marriage, relations with associates, work, clubs, neighborhoods, and places of worship. They may be regulated by law, custom, or mutual agreement, and are the basis of social groups and society as a whole.

A relationship is normally viewed as a connection between two individuals, such as a romantic or intimate relationship, or a parent–child relationship. Individuals can also have relationships with groups of people, such as the relation between a pastor and his congregation, an uncle and a family, or a mayor and a town. Finally, groups or even nations may have relations with each other, though this is a much broader domain than that covered under the topic of interpersonal relationships. See such articles as international relations for more information on associations between groups. Most scholarly work on relationships focuses on the small subset of interpersonal relationships involving romantic partners in pairs or dyads.

Interpersonal relationships usually involve some level of interdependence. People in a relationship tend to influence each other, share their thoughts and feelings, and engage in activities together. Because of this interdependence, most things that change or impact one member of the relationship will have some level of impact on the other member.[1] The study of interpersonal relationships involves several branches of the social sciences, including such disciplines as sociology, psychology, anthropology, and social work. The scientific study of relationships is referred to as relationship science and distinguishes itself from anecdotal evidence or pseudo-experts by basing conclusions on data and objective analysis. Interpersonal ties are also a subject in mathematical sociology.

Development

Interpersonal relationships are dynamic systems that change continuously during their existence. Like living organisms, relationships have a beginning, a lifespan, and an end. They tend to grow and improve gradually, as people get to know each other and become closer emotionally, or they gradually deteriorate as people drift apart, move on with their lives and form new relationships with others. One of the most influential models of relationship development was proposed by psychologist George Levinger.[2] This model was formulated to describe heterosexual, adult romantic relationships, but it has been applied to other kinds of interpersonal relations as well. According to the model, the natural development of a relationship follows five stages:

1. *Acquaintance* – Becoming acquainted depends on previous relationships, physical proximity, first impressions, and a variety of other factors. If two people begin to like each other, continued interactions may lead to the next stage, but acquaintance can continue indefinitely.
2. *Buildup* – During this stage, people begin to trust and care about each other. The need for intimacy, compatibility and such filtering agents as common background and goals will influence whether or not interaction continues.
3. *Continuation* – This stage follows a mutual commitment to a long-term friendship, romantic relationship, or marriage. It is generally a long, relative stable period. Nevertheless, continued growth and development will occur during this time. Mutual trust is important for sustaining the relationship.
4. *Deterioration* – Not all relationships deteriorate, but those that do tend to show signs of trouble. Boredom, resentment, and dissatisfaction may occur, and individuals may communicate less and avoid self-disclosure. Loss of trust and betrayals may take place as the downward spiral continues, eventually ending the relationship. (Alternately, the participants may find some way to resolve the problems and reestablish trust.)
5. *Termination* – The final stage marks the end of the relationship, either by death in the case of a healthy relationship, or by separation.

Friendships may involve some degree of transitivity. In other words, a person may become a friend of an existing friend's friend. However, if two people have a sexual relationship with the same person, they may become competitors rather than friends. Accordingly, sexual behavior with the sexual partner of a friend may damage the friendship (see love triangle). Sexual activities between two friends tend to alter that relationship, either by "taking it to the next level" or by severing it.

Flourishing relationships

Positive psychologists use the term "flourishing relationships" to describe interpersonal relationships that are not merely happy, but instead characterized by intimacy, growth, and resilience.[3] Flourishing relationships also allow a dynamic balance between focus on the intimate relationships and focus on other social relationships.

Background

While traditional psychologists specializing in close relationships have focused on relationship dysfunction, positive psychology argues that relationship health is not merely the absence of relationship dysfunction.[4] Healthy relationships are built on a foundation of secure attachment and are maintained with love and purposeful positive relationship behaviors. Additionally, healthy relationships can be made to "flourish." Positive psychologists are exploring what makes existing relationships flourish and what skills can be taught to partners to enhance their existing and future personal relationships. A social skills approach posits that individuals differ in their degree of communication skill, which has implications for their relationships. Relationships in which partners possess and enact relevant communication skills are more satisfying and stable than relationships in which partners lack appropriate communication skills. [5]

Adult attachment

Healthy relationships are built on a foundation of secure attachments. Adult attachment models represent an internal set of expectations and preferences regarding relationship intimacy that guide behavior.[4] Secure adult attachment, characterized by low attachment-related avoidance and anxiety, has numerous benefits. Within the context of safe, secure attachments, people can pursue optimal human functioning and flourishing.[4]

Love

The capacity for love gives depth to human relationships, brings people closer to each other physically and emotionally, and makes people think expansively about themselves and the world.[4] In his triangular theory of love, psychologist Robert Sternberg theorizes that love is a mix of three components: some (1) passion, or physical attraction; (2) intimacy, or feelings of closeness; and (3) commitment, involving the decision to initiate and sustain a relationship. The presence of all three components characterizes consummate love, the most durable type of love. In addition, the presence of intimacy and passion in marital relationships predicts marital satisfaction. Also, commitment is the best predictor of relationship satisfaction, especially in long-term relationships. Positive consequences of being in love include increased self-esteem and self-efficacy.[4]

Theories and empirical research

Confucianism

Confucianism is a study and theory of relationships especially within hierarchies.[6] Social harmony — the central goal of Confucianism — results in part from every individual knowing his or her place in the social order, and playing his or her part well. Particular duties arise from each person's particular situation in relation to others. The individual stands simultaneously in several different relationships with different people: as a junior in relation to parents and elders, and as a senior in relation to younger siblings, students, and others. Juniors are considered in Confucianism to owe their seniors reverence and seniors have duties of benevolence and concern toward juniors. A focus on mutuality is prevalent in East Asian cultures to this day.

Minding relationships

The mindfulness theory of relationships shows how closeness in relationships may be enhanced. Minding is the "reciprocal knowing process involving the nonstop, interrelated thoughts, feelings, and behaviors of persons in a relationship."[7] Five components of "minding" include:[4]

1. Knowing and being known: seeking to understand the partner
2. Making relationship-enhancing attributions for behaviors: giving the benefit of the doubt
3. Accepting and respecting: empathy and social skills
4. Maintaining reciprocity: active participation in relationship enhancement
5. Continuity in minding: persisting in mindfulness

Culture of appreciation

After studying married couples for many years, psychologist John Gottman has proposed the theory of the "magic ratio" for successful marriages. The theory says that for a marriage to be successful, couples must average a ratio of five positive interactions to one negative interaction. As the ratio moves to 1:1, divorce becomes more likely.[4] Interpersonal interactions associated with negative relationships include criticism, contempt, defensiveness, and stonewalling. Over time, therapy aims to turn these interpersonal strategies into more positive ones, which include complaint, appreciation, acceptance of responsibility, and self-soothing. Similarly, partners in interpersonal relationships can incorporate positive components into difficult subjects in order to avoid emotional disconnection. Knowing when to go to the next step is very important.

Capitalizing on positive events

People can capitalize on positive events in an interpersonal context to work toward flourishing relationships. People often turn to others to share their good news (termed "capitalization"). Studies show that both the act of telling others about good events and the response of the person with whom the event was shared have personal and interpersonal consequences, including increased positive emotions, subjective well-being, and self-esteem, and relationship benefits including intimacy, commitment, trust, liking, closeness, and stability.[8] Studies show that the act of communicating positive events was associated with increased positive affect and well-being (beyond the impact of the positive event itself ε). Other studies have found that relationships in which partners responded to "good news" communication enthusiastically were associated with higher relationship well-being.[9]

Other perspectives

Neurobiology of interpersonal connections

There is an emerging body of research across multiple disciplines investigating the neurological basis of attachment and the prosocial emotions and behaviors that are the prerequisites for healthy adult relationships.[4] The social environment, mediated by attachment, influences the maturation of structures in a child's brain. This might explain how infant attachment affects adult emotional health. Researchers are currently investigating the link between positive caregiver–child relationships and the development of hormone systems, such as the HPA axis.

Applications

Researchers are developing an approach to couples therapy that moves partners from patterns of repeated conflict to patterns of more positive, comfortable exchanges. Goals of therapy include development of social and interpersonal skills. Expressing gratitude and sharing appreciation for a partner is the primary means for creating a positive relationship. Positive marital counseling also emphasizes mindfulness. The further study of "flourishing relationships could shape the future of premarital and marital counseling as well."[4]

Controversies

Some researchers criticize positive psychology for studying positive processes in isolation from negative processes. Positive psychologists argue that positive and negative processes in relationships may be better understood as functionally independent not as opposites of each other.[10]

See also

- Intimate relationship
- Interpersonal attraction
- Outline of relationships

References

[1] Berscheid, E., & Peplau, L.A. (1983). The emerging science of relationships. In H.H. Kelley, et al. (Eds.), *Close relationships*. (pp. 1–19). New York: W.H. Freeman and Company.

[2] Levinger, G. (1983). Development and change. In H.H. Kelley, et al. (Eds.), *Close relationships*. (pp. 315–359). New York: W.H. Freeman and Company.

[3] Fincham, F.D., & Beach, S.R.H. (2010). Of memes and marriage: Toward a positive relationship science. *Journal of Family Theory & Review*, 2, 4–24.

[4] Snyder, C.R., & Lopez, Shane, J. (2007). "Positive psychology: the scientific and practical explorations of human strengths.", Thousand Oaks, California: Sage Publications, 297–321.

[5] Burleson; Samter (April-June 2009). *Communication Quarterly* **57** (2).

[6] Richey, Jeff (2011 [last update]). "Confucius" (http://www.iep.utm.edu/confuciu/). *iep.utm.edu*. Internet Encyclopedia of Philosophy. . Retrieved August 11, 2011.

[7] John H. Harvey, J.H., & Pauwels, B.G. (2009). Relationship Connection: A Redux on the Role of Minding and the Quality of Feeling Special in the Enhancement of Closeness. [Eds.] Snyder, C.D., & Lopez, S.J. *Oxford Handbook of Positive Psychology: Second Edition*. Oxford: Oxford University Press. 385–392.

[8] Gable, S.L., & Reis, H.T. (2010). Good News! Capitalizing on Positive Events in an Interpersonal Context. *Advances in Experimental Social Psychology*, 42, 195–257.

[9] Gable, S.L., Reis, H.T., Impett, E.A., Asher, E.R. (2004). What Do You Do When Things Go Right? The Intrapersonal and Interpersonal Benefits of Sharing Positive Events. *Journal of Personality and Social Psychology*, 87, 228–245.

[10] Maniaci, M.R., & Reis, H.T. (2010). The Marriage of Positive Psychology and Relationship Science: A Reply to Fincham and Beach. *Journal of Family Theory & Review*, 2, 47–53.

Gene

A **gene** is a molecular unit of heredity of a living organism. It is a name given to some stretches of DNA and RNA that code for a polypeptide or for an RNA chain that has a function in the organism. Living beings depend on genes, as they specify all proteins and functional RNA chains. Genes hold the information to build and maintain an organism's cells and pass genetic traits to offspring, although some organelles (e.g. mitochondria) are self-replicating and are not coded for by the organism's DNA. All organisms have many genes corresponding to various biological traits, some of which are immediately visible, such as eye color or number of limbs, and some of which are not, such as blood type or increased risk for specific diseases, or the thousands of basic biochemical processes that comprise life.

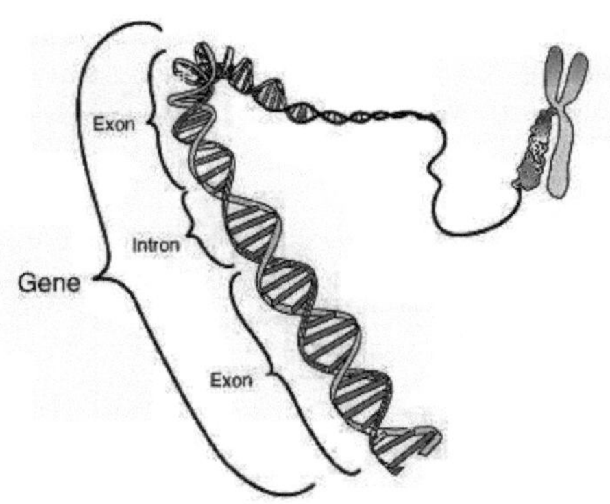

This stylistic diagram shows a gene in relation to the double helix structure of DNA and to a chromosome (right). The chromosome is X-shaped because it is dividing. Introns are regions often found in eukaryote genes that are removed in the splicing process (after the DNA is transcribed into RNA): Only the exons encode the protein. This diagram labels a region of only 50 or so bases as a gene. In reality, most genes are hundreds of times larger.

A modern working definition of a gene is "*a locatable region of genomic sequence, corresponding to a unit of inheritance, which is associated with regulatory regions, transcribed regions, and or other functional sequence regions* ".[1] [2] Colloquial usage of the term *gene* (e.g. "good genes", "hair color gene") may actually refer to an allele: a *gene* is the basic instruction—a sequence of nucleic acids (DNA or, in the case of certain viruses RNA), while an *allele* is one variant of that gene. Referring to having a gene for a trait is no longer the scientifically accepted usage. In most cases, all people would have a gene for the trait in question, but certain people will have a specific allele of that gene, which results in the trait variant. Further, genes code for proteins, which might result in identifiable traits, but it is the gene, not the trait, which is inherited.

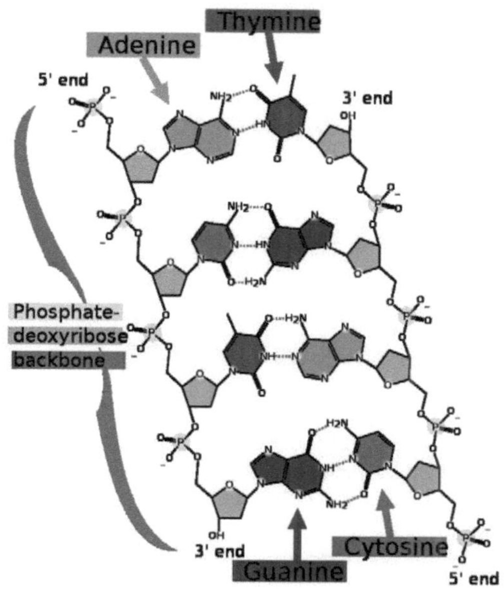

The chemical structure of a four-base fragment of a DNA double helix.

Physical definitions

RNA genes and genomes

When proteins are manufactured, the gene is first copied into RNA as an intermediate product. In other cases, the RNA molecules are the actual functional products. For example, RNAs known as ribozymes are capable of enzymatic function, and microRNA has a regulatory role. The DNA sequences from which such RNAs are transcribed are known as RNA genes.

Some viruses store their entire genomes in the form of RNA, and contain no DNA at all. Because they use RNA to store genes, their cellular hosts may synthesize their proteins as soon as they are infected and without the delay in waiting for transcription. On the other hand, RNA retroviruses, such as HIV, require the reverse transcription of their genome from RNA into DNA before their proteins can be synthesized. In 2006, French researchers came across a puzzling example of RNA-mediated inheritance in mice. Mice with a loss-of-function mutation in the gene Kit have white tails. Offspring of these mutants can have white tails despite having only normal Kit genes. The research team traced this effect back to mutated Kit RNA.[3] While RNA is common as genetic storage material in viruses, in mammals in particular RNA inheritance has been observed very rarely.

Functional structure of a gene

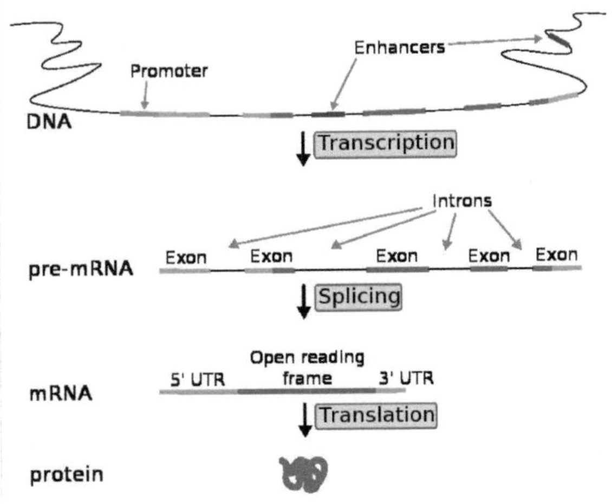

Diagram of the "typical" eukaryotic protein-coding **gene**. Promoters and enhancers determine what portions of the DNA will be transcribed into the precursor mRNA (pre-mRNA). The pre-mRNA is then spliced into messenger RNA (mRNA) which is later translated into protein.

The vast majority of living organisms encode their genes in long strands of DNA. DNA (deoxyribonucleic acid) consists of a chain made from four types of nucleotide subunits, each composed of: a five-carbon sugar (2'-deoxyribose), a phosphate group, and one of the four bases adenine, cytosine, guanine, and thymine. The most common form of DNA in a cell is in a double helix structure, in which two individual DNA strands twist around each other in a right-handed spiral. In this structure, the base pairing rules specify that guanine pairs with cytosine and adenine pairs with thymine. The base pairing between guanine and cytosine forms three hydrogen bonds, whereas the base pairing between adenine and thymine forms two hydrogen bonds. The two strands in a double helix must therefore be *complementary*, that is, their bases must align such that the adenines of one strand are paired with the thymines of the other strand, and so on.

Due to the chemical composition of the pentose residues of the bases, DNA strands have directionality. One end of a DNA polymer contains an exposed hydroxyl group on the deoxyribose; this is known as the 3' end of the molecule. The other end contains an exposed phosphate group; this is the 5' end. The directionality of DNA is vitally important to many cellular processes, since double helices are necessarily directional (a strand running 5'-3' pairs with a complementary strand running 3'-5'), and processes such as DNA replication occur in only one direction. All nucleic acid synthesis in a cell occurs in the 5'-3' direction, because new monomers are added via a dehydration reaction that uses the exposed 3' hydroxyl as a nucleophile.

The expression of genes encoded in DNA begins by transcribing the gene into RNA, a second type of nucleic acid that is very similar to DNA, but whose monomers contain the sugar ribose rather than deoxyribose. RNA also contains the base uracil in place of thymine. RNA molecules are less stable than DNA and are typically single-stranded. Genes that encode proteins are composed of a series of three-nucleotide sequences called codons, which serve as the *words* in the genetic *language*. The genetic code specifies the correspondence during protein translation between codons and amino acids. The genetic code is nearly the same for all known organisms.

All genes have regulatory regions in addition to regions that explicitly code for a protein or RNA product. A regulatory region shared by almost all genes is known as the promoter, which provides a position that is recognized by the transcription machinery when a gene is about to be transcribed and expressed. A gene can have more than one promoter, resulting in RNAs that differ in how far they extend in the 5' end.[4] Although promoter regions have a consensus sequence that is the most common sequence at this position, some genes have "strong" promoters that bind the transcription machinery well, and others have "weak" promoters that bind poorly. These weak promoters usually permit a lower rate of transcription than the strong promoters, because the transcription machinery binds to them and initiates transcription less frequently. Other possible regulatory regions include enhancers, which can compensate for a weak promoter. Most regulatory regions are "upstream"—that is, before or toward the 5' end of the transcription initiation site. Eukaryotic promoter regions are much more complex and difficult to identify than prokaryotic promoters.

Many prokaryotic genes are organized into operons, or groups of genes whose products have related functions and which are transcribed as a unit. By contrast, eukaryotic genes are transcribed only one at a time, but may include long stretches of DNA called introns which are transcribed but never translated into protein (they are spliced out before translation). Splicing can also occur in prokaryotic genes, but is less common than in eukaryotes.[5]

Chromosomes

The total complement of genes in an organism or cell is known as its genome, which may be stored on one or more chromosomes; the region of the chromosome at which a particular gene is located is called its locus. A chromosome consists of a single, very long DNA helix on which thousands of genes are encoded. Prokaryotes—bacteria and archaea—typically store their genomes on a single large, circular chromosome, sometimes supplemented by additional small circles of DNA called plasmids, which usually encode only a few genes and are easily transferable between individuals. For example, the genes for antibiotic resistance are usually encoded on bacterial plasmids and can be passed between individual cells, even those of different species, via horizontal gene transfer. Although some simple eukaryotes also possess plasmids with small numbers of genes, the majority of eukaryotic genes are stored on multiple linear chromosomes, which are packed within the nucleus in complex with storage proteins called histones. The manner in which DNA is stored on the histone, as well as chemical modifications of the histone itself, are regulatory mechanisms governing whether a particular region of DNA is accessible for gene expression. The ends of eukaryotic chromosomes are capped by long stretches of repetitive sequences called telomeres, which do not code for any gene product but are present to prevent degradation of coding and regulatory regions during DNA replication. The length of the telomeres tends to decrease each time the genome is replicated in preparation for cell division; the loss of telomeres has been proposed as an explanation for cellular senescence, or the loss of the ability to divide, and by extension for the aging process in organisms.[6]

Whereas the chromosomes of prokaryotes are relatively gene-dense, those of eukaryotes often contain so-called "junk DNA", or regions of DNA that serve no obvious function. Simple single-celled eukaryotes have relatively small amounts of such DNA, whereas the genomes of complex multicellular organisms, including humans, contain an absolute majority of DNA without an identified function.[7] However it now appears that, although protein-coding DNA makes up barely 2% of the human genome, about 80% of the bases in the genome may be expressed, so the term "junk DNA" may be a misnomer.[2]

Gene expression

In all organisms, there are two major steps separating a protein-coding gene from its protein: First, the DNA on which the gene resides must be *transcribed* from DNA to messenger RNA (mRNA); and, second, it must be *translated* from mRNA to protein. RNA-coding genes must still go through the first step, but are not translated into protein. The process of producing a biologically functional molecule of either RNA or protein is called gene expression, and the resulting molecule itself is called a gene product.

Genetic code

The genetic code is the set of rules by which a gene is translated into a functional protein. Each gene consists of a specific sequence of nucleotides encoded in a DNA (or sometimes RNA in some viruses[8]) strand; a correspondence between nucleotides, the basic building blocks of genetic material, and amino acids, the basic building blocks of proteins, must be established for genes to be successfully translated into functional proteins. Sets of three nucleotides, known as codons, each correspond to a specific amino acid or to a signal; three codons are known as "stop codons" and, instead of specifying a new amino acid, alert the translation machinery that the end of the gene has been reached. There are 64 possible codons (four possible nucleotides at each of three positions, hence 4^3 possible codons) and only 20 standard amino acids; hence the code is redundant and multiple codons can specify the same amino acid. The correspondence between codons and amino acids is nearly universal among all known living organisms.

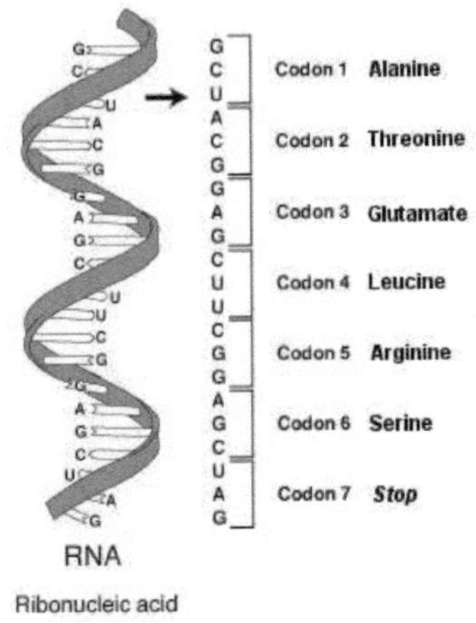

Schematic diagram of a single-stranded RNA molecule illustrating the position of three-base codons.

Transcription

The process of genetic transcription produces a single-stranded RNA molecule known as messenger RNA, whose nucleotide sequence is complementary to the DNA from which it was transcribed. The DNA strand whose sequence matches that of the RNA is known as the coding strand and the strand from which the RNA was synthesized is the template strand. Transcription is performed by an enzyme called an RNA polymerase, which reads the template strand in the 3' to 5' direction and synthesizes the RNA from 5' to 3'. To initiate transcription, the polymerase first recognizes and binds a promoter region of the gene. Thus a major mechanism of gene regulation is the blocking or sequestering of the promoter region, either by tight binding by repressor molecules that physically block the polymerase, or by organizing the DNA so that the promoter region is not accessible.

In prokaryotes, transcription occurs in the cytoplasm; for very long transcripts, translation may begin at the 5' end of the RNA while the 3' end is still being transcribed. In eukaryotes, transcription necessarily occurs in the nucleus, where the cell's DNA is sequestered; the RNA molecule produced by the polymerase is known as the primary transcript and must undergo post-transcriptional modifications before being exported to the cytoplasm for translation. The splicing of introns present within the transcribed region is a modification unique to eukaryotes; alternative splicing mechanisms can result in mature transcripts from the same gene having different sequences and thus coding for different proteins. This is a major form of regulation in eukaryotic cells.

Translation

Translation is the process by which a mature mRNA molecule is used as a template for synthesizing a new protein. Translation is carried out by ribosomes, large complexes of RNA and protein responsible for carrying out the chemical reactions to add new amino acids to a growing polypeptide chain by the formation of peptide bonds. The genetic code is read three nucleotides at a time, in units called codons, via interactions with specialized RNA molecules called transfer RNA (tRNA). Each tRNA has three unpaired bases known as the anticodon that are complementary to the codon it reads; the tRNA is also covalently attached to the amino acid specified by the complementary codon. When the tRNA binds to its complementary codon in an mRNA strand, the ribosome ligates its amino acid cargo to the new polypeptide chain, which is synthesized from amino terminus to carboxyl terminus. During and after its synthesis, the new protein must fold to its active three-dimensional structure before it can carry out its cellular function.

DNA replication and inheritance

The growth, development, and reproduction of organisms relies on cell division, or the process by which a single cell divides into two usually identical daughter cells. This requires first making a duplicate copy of every gene in the genome in a process called DNA replication. The copies are made by specialized enzymes known as DNA polymerases, which "read" one strand of the double-helical DNA, known as the template strand, and synthesize a new complementary strand. Because the DNA double helix is held together by base pairing, the sequence of one strand completely specifies the sequence of its complement; hence only one strand needs to be read by the enzyme to produce a faithful copy. The process of DNA replication is semiconservative; that is, the copy of the genome inherited by each daughter cell contains one original and one newly synthesized strand of DNA.[9]

After DNA replication is complete, the cell must physically separate the two copies of the genome and divide into two distinct membrane-bound cells. In prokaryotes - bacteria and archaea - this usually occurs via a relatively simple process called binary fission, in which each circular genome attaches to the cell membrane and is separated into the daughter cells as the membrane invaginates to split the cytoplasm into two membrane-bound portions. Binary fission is extremely fast compared to the rates of cell division in eukaryotes. Eukaryotic cell division is a more complex process known as the cell cycle; DNA replication occurs during a phase of this cycle known as S phase, whereas the process of segregating chromosomes and splitting the cytoplasm occurs during M phase. In many single-celled eukaryotes such as yeast, reproduction by budding is common, which results in asymmetrical portions of cytoplasm in the two daughter cells.

Molecular inheritance

The duplication and transmission of genetic material from one generation of cells to the next is the basis for molecular inheritance, and the link between the classical and molecular pictures of genes. Organisms inherit the characteristics of their parents because the cells of the offspring contain copies of the genes in their parents' cells. In asexually reproducing organisms, the offspring will be a genetic copy or clone of the parent organism. In sexually reproducing organisms, a specialized form of cell division called meiosis produces cells called gametes or germ cells that are haploid, or contain only one copy of each gene. The gametes produced by females are called eggs or ova, and those produced by males are called sperm. Two gametes fuse to form a fertilized egg, a single cell that once again has a diploid number of genes—each with one copy from the mother and one copy from the father.

During the process of meiotic cell division, an event called genetic recombination or *crossing-over* can sometimes occur, in which a length of DNA on one chromatid is swapped with a length of DNA on the corresponding sister chromatid. This has no effect if the alleles on the chromatids are the same, but results in reassortment of otherwise linked alleles if they are different. The Mendelian principle of independent assortment asserts that each of a parent's two genes for each trait will sort independently into gametes; which allele an organism inherits for one trait is unrelated to which allele it inherits for another trait. This is in fact only true for genes that do not reside on the same chromosome, or are located very far from one another on the same chromosome. The closer two genes lie on the same chromosome, the more closely they will be associated in gametes and the more often they will appear together; genes that are very close are essentially never separated because it is extremely unlikely that a crossover point will occur between them. This is known as genetic linkage.

History

The notion of a gene[10] is evolving with the science of genetics, which began when Gregor Mendel noticed that biological variations are inherited from parent organisms as specific, discrete traits. The biological entity responsible for defining traits was later termed a *gene*, but the biological basis for inheritance remained unknown until DNA was identified as the genetic material in the 1940s. Prior to Mendel's work, the dominant theory of heredity was one of blending inheritance, which proposes that the traits of the parents blend or mix in a smooth, continuous gradient in the offspring. Although Mendel's work was largely unrecognized after its first publication in 1866, it was rediscovered in 1900 by three European scientists, Hugo de Vries, Carl Correns, and Erich von Tschermak, who had reached similar conclusions from their own research. However, these scientists were not yet aware of the identity of the 'discrete units' on which genetic material resides.

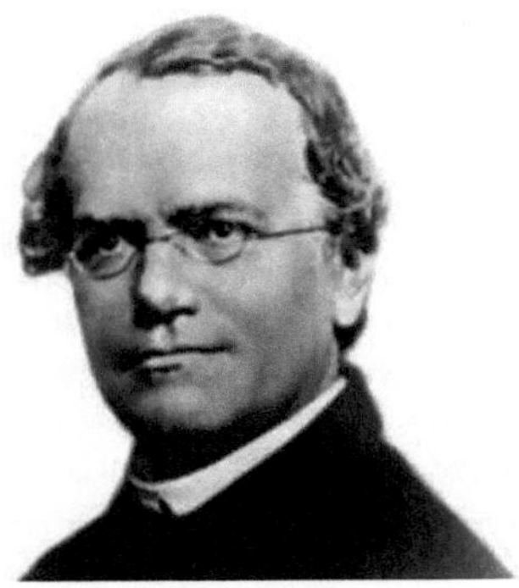

Gregor Mendel

The existence of genes was first suggested by Gregor Mendel (1822–1884), who, in the 1860s, studied inheritance in peaplants (*Pisum sativum*) and hypothesized a factor that conveys traits from parent to offspring. He spent over 10 years of his life on one experiment. Although he did not use the term *gene*, he explained his results in terms of inherited characteristics. Mendel was also the first to hypothesize independent assortment, the distinction between dominant and recessive traits, the distinction between a heterozygote and homozygote, and the difference between what would later be described as genotype (the genetic material of an organism) and phenotype (the visible traits of that organism).

Charles Darwin used the term Gemmule to describe a microscopic unit of inheritance, and what would later become known as Chromosomes had been observed separating out during cell division by Wilhelm Hofmeister as early as 1848. The idea that chromosomes are the carriers of inheritance was expressed in 1883 by Wilhelm Roux. Darwin also coined the word *pangenesis* by (1868).[11] The word pangenesis is made from the Greek words *pan* (a prefix meaning "whole", "encompassing") and *genesis* ("birth") or *genos* ("origin").

Mendel's concept was given a name by Hugo de Vries in 1889, in his book *Intracellular Pangenesis*; although probably unaware of Mendel's work at the time, he coined the term "pangen" for "the smallest particle [representing] one hereditary characteristic".[12] Danish botanist Wilhelm Johannsen coined the word "gene" ("gen" in Danish and German) in 1909 to describe the fundamental physical and functional units of heredity,[13] while the related word genetics was first used by William Bateson in 1905.[14] He derived the word from de Vries' "pangen". In the early 1900s, Mendel's work received renewed attention from scientists. In 1910, Thomas Hunt Morgan showed that genes reside on specific chromosomes. He later showed that genes occupy specific locations on the chromosome. With this knowledge, Morgan and his students began the first chromosomal map of the fruit fly *Drosophila*. In 1928, Frederick Griffith showed that genes could be transferred. In what is now known as Griffith's experiment, injections into a mouse of a deadly strain of bacteria that had been heat-killed transferred genetic information to a safe strain of the same bacteria, killing the mouse.

A series of subsequent discoveries led to the realization decades later that chromosomes within cells are the carriers of genetic material, and that they are made of DNA (deoxyribonucleic acid), a polymeric molecule found in all cells on which the 'discrete units' of Mendelian inheritance are encoded. In 1941, George Wells Beadle and Edward Lawrie Tatum showed that mutations in genes caused errors in specific steps in metabolic pathways. This showed that specific genes code for specific proteins, leading to the "one gene, one enzyme" hypothesis.[14] Oswald Avery, Colin Munro MacLeod, and Maclyn McCarty showed in 1944 that DNA holds the gene's information.[15] In 1953,

James D. Watson and Francis Crick demonstrated the molecular structure of DNA. Together, these discoveries established the central dogma of molecular biology, which states that proteins are translated from RNA which is transcribed from DNA. This dogma has since been shown to have exceptions, such as reverse transcription in retroviruses.

In 1972, Walter Fiers and his team at the Laboratory of Molecular Biology of the University of Ghent (Ghent, Belgium) were the first to determine the sequence of a gene: the gene for Bacteriophage MS2 coat protein.[16] Richard J. Roberts and Phillip Sharp discovered in 1977 that genes can be split into segments. This led to the idea that one gene can make several proteins. Recently (as of 2003–2006), biological results let the notion of gene appear more slippery. In particular, genes do not seem to sit side by side on DNA like discrete beads. Instead, regions of the DNA producing distinct proteins may overlap, so that the idea emerges that "genes are one long continuum".[1] It was first hypothesized in 1986 by Walter Gilbert that neither DNA nor protein would be required in such a primitive system as that of a very early stage of the earth if RNA could perform as simply a catalyst and genetic information storage processor.

The modern study of genetics at the level of DNA is known as molecular genetics and the synthesis of molecular genetics with traditional Darwinian evolution is known as the modern evolutionary synthesis.

Mendelian inheritance and classical genetics

According to the theory of Mendelian inheritance, variations in phenotype—the observable physical and behavioral characteristics of an organism—are due to variations in genotype, or the organism's particular set of genes, each of which specifies a particular trait. Different forms of a gene, which may give rise to different phenotypes, are known as alleles. Organisms such as the pea plants Mendel worked on, along with many plants and animals, have two alleles for each trait, one inherited from each parent. Alleles may be dominant or recessive; dominant alleles give rise to their corresponding phenotypes when paired with any other allele for the same trait, whereas recessive alleles give rise to their corresponding phenotype only when paired with another copy of the same allele. For example, if the allele specifying tall stems in pea plants is dominant over the allele specifying short stems, then pea plants that inherit one tall allele from one parent and one short allele from the other parent will also have tall stems. Mendel's work demonstrated that alleles assort independently in the production of gametes, or germ cells, ensuring variation in the next generation.

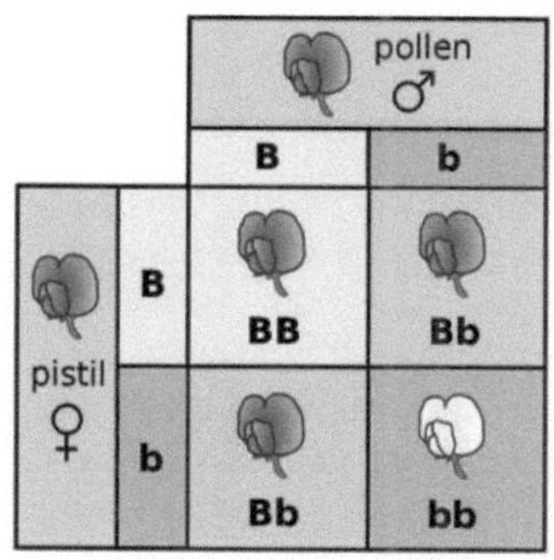

Crossing between two pea plants heterozygous for purple (B, dominant) and white (b, recessive) blossoms

Mutation

DNA replication is for the most part extremely accurate, with an error rate per site of around 10^{-6} to 10^{-10} in eukaryotes.[9] Rare, spontaneous alterations in the base sequence of a particular gene arise from a number of sources, such as errors in DNA replication and the aftermath of DNA damage. These errors are called mutations. The cell contains many DNA repair mechanisms for preventing mutations and maintaining the integrity of the genome; however, in some cases—such as breaks in both DNA strands of a chromosome—repairing the physical damage to the molecule is a higher priority than producing an exact copy. Due to the degeneracy of the genetic code, some mutations in protein-coding genes are *silent*, or produce no change in the amino acid sequence of the protein for which they code; for example, the codons UCU and UUC both code for serine, so the U↔C mutation has no effect on the protein. Mutations that do have phenotypic effects are most often neutral or deleterious to the organism, but sometimes they confer benefits to the organism's fitness.

Mutations propagated to the next generation lead to variations within a species' population. Variants of a single gene are known as alleles, and differences in alleles may give rise to differences in traits. Although it is rare for the variants in a single gene to have clearly distinguishable phenotypic effects, certain well-defined traits are in fact controlled by single genetic loci. A gene's most common allele is called the wild type allele, and rare alleles are called mutants. However, this does not imply that the wild-type allele is the ancestor from which the mutants are descended.

Genome

Chromosomal organization

The total complement of genes in an organism or cell is known as its genome. In prokaryotes, the vast majority of genes are located on a single chromosome of circular DNA, while eukaryotes usually possess multiple individual linear DNA helices packed into dense DNA-protein complexes called chromosomes. Genes that appear together on one chromosome of one species may appear on separate chromosomes in another species. Many species carry more than one copy of their genome within each of their somatic cells. Cells or organisms with only one copy of each chromosome are called haploid; those with two copies are called diploid; and those with more than two copies are called polyploid. The copies of genes on the chromosomes are not necessarily identical. In sexually reproducing organisms, one copy is normally inherited from each parent.

Number of genes

Early estimates of the number of human genes that used expressed sequence tag data put it at 50 000–100 000.[18] Following the sequencing of the human genome and other genomes, it has been found that rather few genes (~20 000 in human, mouse and fly, ~13 000 in roundworm, >46 000 in rice) encode all the proteins in an organism.[19] These protein-coding sequences make up 1–2% of the human genome.[20] A large part of the genome is transcribed however, to introns, retrotransposons and seemingly a large array of noncoding RNAs.[19] [20] Total number of proteins (the Earth's proteome) is estimated to be 5 million sequences.[21]

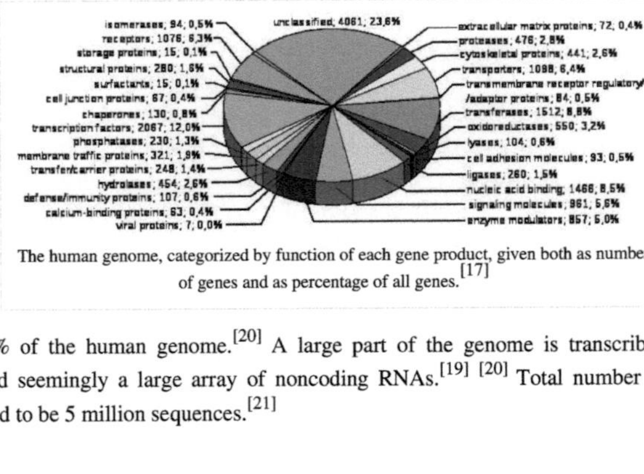

The human genome, categorized by function of each gene product, given both as number of genes and as percentage of all genes.[17]

Genetic and genomic nomenclature

Gene nomenclature has been established by the HUGO Gene Nomenclature Committee (HGNC) for each known human gene in the form of an approved gene name and symbol (short-form abbreviation). All approved symbols are stored in the HGNC Database [22]. Each symbol is unique and each gene is only given one approved gene symbol. This also facilitates electronic data retrieval from publications. In preference each symbol maintains parallel construction in different members of a gene family and can be used in other species, especially the mouse.

Evolutionary concept of a gene

George C. Williams first explicitly advocated the gene-centric view of evolution in his 1966 book *Adaptation and Natural Selection*. He proposed an evolutionary concept of gene to be used when we are talking about natural selection favoring some genes. The definition is: "that which segregates and recombines with appreciable frequency." According to this definition, even an asexual genome could be considered a gene, insofar that it have an appreciable permanency through many generations.

The difference is: the molecular gene *transcribes* as a unit, and the evolutionary gene *inherits* as a unit.

Richard Dawkins' books *The Selfish Gene* (1976) and *The Extended Phenotype* (1982) defended the idea that the gene is the only replicator in living systems. This means that only genes transmit their structure largely intact and are potentially immortal in the form of copies. So, genes should be the unit of selection. In *The Selfish Gene* Dawkins attempts to redefine the word 'gene' to mean "an inheritable unit" instead of the generally accepted definition of "a section of DNA coding for a particular protein". In *River Out of Eden*, Dawkins further refined the idea of gene-centric selection by describing life as a river of compatible genes flowing through geological time. Scoop up a bucket of genes from the river of genes, and we have an organism serving as temporary bodies or survival machines. A river of genes may fork into two branches representing two non-interbreeding species as a result of geographical separation.

Gene targeting and implications

Gene targeting is commonly referred to techniques for altering or disrupting mouse genes and provides the mouse models for studying the roles of individual genes in embryonic development, human disorders, aging and diseases. The mouse models, where one or more of its genes are deactivated or made inoperable, are called knockout mice. Since the first reports in which homologous recombination in embryonic stem cells was used to generate gene-targeted mice,[23] gene targeting has proven to be a powerful means of precisely manipulating the mammalian genome, producing at least ten thousand mutant mouse strains and it is now possible to introduce mutations that can be activated at specific time points, or in specific cells or organs, both during development and in the adult animal.[24] [25]

Gene targeting strategies have been expanded to all kinds of modifications, including point mutations, isoform deletions, mutant allele correction, large pieces of chromosomal DNA insertion and deletion, tissue specific disruption combined with spatial and temporal regulation and so on. It is predicted that the ability to generate mouse models with predictable phenotypes will have a major impact on studies of all phases of development, immunology, neurobiology, oncology, physiology, metabolism, and human diseases. Gene targeting is also in theory applicable to species from which totipotent embryonic stem cells can be established, and therefore may offer a potential to the improvement of domestic animals and plants.[25] [26]

Changing concept

The concept of the gene has changed considerably (see history section). From the original definition of a "unit of inheritance", the term evolved to mean a DNA-based unit that can exert its effects on the organism through RNA or protein products. It was also previously believed that one gene makes one protein; this concept was overthrown by the discovery of alternative splicing and trans-splicing.[14]

The definition of a gene is still changing. The first cases of RNA-based inheritance have been discovered in mammals.[3] Evidence is also accumulating that the control regions of a gene do not necessarily have to be close to the coding sequence on the linear molecule or even on the same chromosome. Spilianakis and colleagues discovered that the promoter region of the interferon-gamma gene on chromosome 10 and the regulatory regions of the T(H)2 cytokine locus on chromosome 11 come into close proximity in the nucleus possibly to be jointly regulated.[27]

The concept that genes are clearly delimited is also being eroded. There is evidence for fused proteins stemming from two adjacent genes that can produce two separate protein products. While it is not clear whether these fusion proteins are functional, the phenomenon is more frequent than previously thought.[28] Even more ground-breaking than the discovery of fused genes is the observation that some proteins can be composed of exons from far away regions and even different chromosomes.[2] [29] This new data has led to an updated, and probably tentative, definition of a gene as "a union of genomic sequences encoding a coherent set of potentially overlapping functional products".[14] This new definition categorizes genes by functional products, whether they be proteins or RNA, rather than specific DNA loci; all regulatory elements of DNA are therefore classified as *gene-associated* regions.[14]

See also

- Big gene
- Copy number variation
- DNA
- Epigenetics
- Full genome sequencing
- Gene-centric view of evolution
- Gene dosage
- Gene expression
- Gene family
- Gene patent
- Gene pool
- Gene redundancy
- Gene therapy
- Genetic algorithm
- Genetic engineering
- Genetics
- Genome
- Genomics
- List of gene prediction software
- List of notable genes
- Meme
- Predictive medicine
- Pseudogene

References

[1] Pearson H (2006). "Genetics: what is a gene?". *Nature* **441** (7092): 398–401. doi:10.1038/441398a. PMID 16724031.

[2] Elizabeth Pennisi (2007). "DNA Study Forces Rethink of What It Means to Be a Gene". *Science* **316** (5831): 1556–1557. doi:10.1126/science.316.5831.1556. PMID 17569836.

[3] Rassoulzadegan M, Grandjean V, Gounon P, Vincent S, Gillot I, Cuzin F (2006). "RNA-mediated non-mendelian inheritance of an epigenetic change in the mouse". *Nature* **441** (7092): 469–74. doi:10.1038/nature04674. PMID 16724059.

[4] Mortazavi A, Williams BA, McCue K, Schaeffer L, Wold B (May 2008). "Mapping and quantifying mammalian transcriptomes by RNA-Seq". *Nat. Methods* **5** (7): 621–8. doi:10.1038/nmeth.1226. PMID 18516045.

[5] Woodson SA (1998). "Ironing out the kinks: splicing and translation in bacteria" (http://genesdev.cshlp.org/content/12/9/1243.full). *Genes Dev.* **12** (9): 1243–7. doi:10.1101/gad.12.9.1243. PMID 9573040. . Retrieved 2009-08-07.

[6] Braig M, Schmitt C (2006). "Oncogene-induced senescence: putting the brakes on tumor development". *Cancer Res* **66** (6): 2881–4. doi:10.1158/0008-5472.CAN-05-4006. PMID 16540631.

[7] International Human Genome Sequencing Consortium (2004). "Finishing the euchromatic sequence of the human genome" (http://www.nature.com/nature/journal/v431/n7011/full/nature03001.html). *Nature* **431** (7011): 931–45. doi:10.1038/nature03001. PMID 15496913. . Retrieved 2009-08-07.

[8] MeSH (2008) National Library of Medicine - Medical Subject Headings. *National library of medicine* http://www.nlm.nih.gov/cgi/mesh/2008/MB_cgi?mode=&term=RNA+Viruses&field=entry (accessed 27 September 2011) B04.820. 19990101.

[9] Watson JD, Baker TA, Bell SP, Gann A, Levine M, Losick R (2004). *Molecular Biology of the Gene* (5th ed.). Peason Benjamin Cummings (Cold Spring Harbor Laboratory Press). ISBN 080534635X.

[10] Error: Bad DOI specified!

[11] Darwin C. (1868). Animals and Plants under Domestication (1868).

[12] Vries, H. de (1889) *Intracellular Pangenesis* (http://www.esp.org/books/devries/pangenesis/facsimile/) ("pangen" definition on page 7 and 40 of this 1910 translation in English)

[13] "The Human Genome Project Timeline" (http://www.genome.gov/25019879). . Retrieved 2006-09-13.

[14] Gerstein Mark B. *et al.* (2007). "What is a gene, post-ENCODE? History and updated definition". *Genome Research* **17** (6): 669–681. doi:10.1101/gr.6339607. PMID 17567988.

[15] Steinman RM, Moberg CL (February 1994). "A triple tribute to the experiment that transformed biology". *J. Exp. Med.* **179** (2): 379–84. doi:10.1084/jem.179.2.379. PMC 2191359. PMID 8294854.

[16] Min Jou W, Haegeman G, Ysebaert M, Fiers W (1972). "Nucleotide sequence of the gene coding for the bacteriophage MS2 coat protein". *Nature* **237** (5350): 82–8. doi:10.1038/237082a0. PMID 4555447.

[17] PANTHER Pie Chart (http://www.pantherdb.org/chart/summary/pantherChart.jsp?filterLevel=1&chartType=1&listType=1&type=5&species=Homo sapiens) at the PANTHER Classification System homepage. Retrieved May 25, 2011

[18] Schuler GD, Boguski MS, Stewart EA, *et al* (October 1996). "A gene map of the human genome" (http://www.sciencemag.org/cgi/content/full/274/5287/540). *Science* **274** (5287): 540–6. doi:10.1126/science.274.5287.540. PMID 8849440. .

[19] Carninci P, Hayashizaki Y (April 2007). "Noncoding RNA transcription beyond annotated genes". *Curr. Opin. Genet. Dev.* **17** (2): 139–44. doi:10.1016/j.gde.2007.02.008. PMID 17317145.

[20] Claverie JM (September 2005). "Fewer genes, more noncoding RNA". *Science* **309** (5740): 1529–30. doi:10.1126/science.1116800. PMID 16141064.

[21] Carolina Perez-Iratxeta, *et al* (2007). "Towards completion of the Earth's proteome" (http://www.nature.com/embor/journal/v8/n12/full/7401117.html). *Nature EMBO reports* **8** (12): 1135–1141. doi:10.1038/sj.embor.7401117. PMC 2267224. PMID 18059312. .

[22] http://www.genenames.org/cgi-bin/hgnc_search.pl

[23] Thomas KR, Capecchi MR. Site-directed mutagenesis by gene targeting in mouse embryo-derived stem cells. Cell. 1987;51:503-12

[24] The 2007 Nobel Prize in Physiology or Medicine - Press Release (http://nobelprize.org/nobel_prizes/medicine/laureates/2007/press.html)

[25] Deng C. In Celebration of Dr. Mario R. Capecchi's Nobel Prize. Int J Biol Sci 2007; 3:417-419. International Journal of Biological Sciences (http://www.biolsci.org/v03p0417.htm)

[26] Mario R. Capecchi (http://www.hhmi.org/research/investigators/capecchi.html)

[27] Spilianakis CG, Lalioti MD, Town T, Lee GR, Flavell RA (June 2005). "Interchromosomal associations between alternatively expressed loci". *Nature* **435** (7042): 637–45. doi:10.1038/nature03574. PMID 15880101.

[28] Parra G, Reymond A, Dabbouseh N, *et al.* (January 2006). "Tandem chimerism as a means to increase protein complexity in the human genome". *Genome Res.* **16** (1): 37–44. doi:10.1101/gr.4145906. PMC 1356127. PMID 16344564.

[29] Kapranov P, Drenkow J, Cheng J, *et al.* (July 2005). "Examples of the complex architecture of the human transcriptome revealed by RACE and high-density tiling arrays". *Genome Res.* **15** (7): 987–97. doi:10.1101/gr.3455305. PMC 1172043. PMID 15998911.

Further reading

- Dawkins, Richard (1990). *The Selfish Gene*. Oxford University Press. ISBN 0-19-286092-5. Google Book Search (http://books.google.com/print?id=WkHO9HI7koEC); first published 1976.
- Dawkins, Richard (1995). *River Out of Eden*. Basic Books. ISBN 0-465-06990-8.
- Ridley, Matt (1999). *Genome: The Autobiography of a Species in 23 Chapters*. Fourth Estate. ISBN 0-00-763573-7.

External links

- Comparative Toxicogenomics Database (http://ctdbase.org/)
- DNA From The Beginning - a primer on genes and DNA (http://www.dnaftb.org/)
- Genes And DNA - Introduction to genes and DNA aimed at non-biologist (http://www.bioinformaticstutorials.com/?p=6)
- Entrez Gene - a searchable database of genes (http://www.ncbi.nlm.nih.gov/sites/entrez?db=gene)
- IDconverter - converts gene IDs between public databases (http://idconverter.bioinfo.cnio.es/)
- iHOP - Information Hyperlinked over Proteins (http://www.ihop-net.org/UniPub/iHOP/)

- TranscriptomeBrowser - Gene expression profile analysis (http://tagc.univ-mrs.fr/tbrowser)
- The Protein Naming Utility, a database to identify and correct deficient gene names (http://www.jcvi.org/pn-utility)
- *Genes* (http://www.mdpi.com/journal/genes/) - an Open Access journal
- IMPC (International Mouse Phenotyping Consortium) (http://www.mousephenotype.org/) - Encyclopedia of mammalian gene function

Foster_care

Foster care is the term used for a system in which a minor who has been made a ward is placed in the private home of a state certified caregiver referred to as a "foster parent".

The state via the family court and child protection agency stand *in loco parentis* to the minor, making all legal decisions while the foster parent is responsible for the day-to-day care of said minor. The foster parent is remunerated by the state for their services.

Foster care is intended to be a short term situation until a permanent placement can be made:[1]

- Reunification with the biological parent(s)
  - When it is deemed in the child's best interest. This is generally the first choice.
- Adoption
  - Preferably by a biological family member such as an aunt or grandparent.
  - If no biological family member is willing or able to adopt, the next preference is for the child to be adopted by the foster parents or by someone else involved in the child's life (such as a teacher or coach). This is to maintain continuity in the child's life.
  - If neither above option are available, the child may be adopted by someone who is a stranger to the child.
- Permanent transfer of guardianship
- If none of these options are viable the plan for the minor may enter OPPLA (Other Planned Permanent Living Arrangement). This option allows the child to stay in custody of the state and the child can stay placed in a foster home, with a relative or a long term care facility (for children with development disabilities, physical disabilities or mental disabilities).

Foster care placement

547,415 children were in publicly supported foster care in the United States in September 2000.[2] In 2009, there were 423,773 children in foster care, a drop of about 20% in a decade.[3]

In 2009, there were about 123,000 children ready for adoptive families in the nation's foster care systems.[4] African American children represented 41% of children in foster care, white children represented 40% and Hispanic children represented 15% in the year 2000.[2]

Children may enter foster care via voluntary or involuntary means. Voluntary placement may occur when a biological parent or lawful guardian is unable to care for a child. Involuntary placement occurs when a child is removed from their biological parent or lawful guardian due to the risk or actual occurrence of physical or psychological harm. In the US, most children enter foster care due to neglect.[5] If a biological parent or lawful guardian is unwilling to care for a child, the child is deemed to be dependent and is placed under the care of the child protection agency.

Regulation, administration, and oversight

The policies regarding foster care as well as the criteria to be met in order to become a foster parent vary according to legal jurisdiction.

In the United States, foster home licensing requirements vary from state to state,but are generally overseen by each state's Department of Social Services or Human Services. In some states, counties have this responsibility. Each state's services are monitored by the federal Department of Health and Human Services through reviews such as Child and Family Services Reviews, Title IV-E Foster Care Eligibility Reviews, Adoption and Foster Care Analysis and Reporting System and Statewide Automated Child Welfare Information System Assessment Reviews.[6]

The foster parent licensing process is often similar to the process to become licensed to adopt. It requires preparation classes as well as an application process. The application varies but may include: a minimum age, verification that your income allows you to meet your expenses, a criminal record check at local, state and federal levels including finger printing and no prior record of child abuse or neglect; a reference from a doctor to ensure that all household members are free from diseases that a child could catch and in sufficient health to parent a child and; letters of reference from an employer and others who know them.

Children found to be unable to function in a foster home may be placed in Residential Treatment Centers (RTCs) or other such group homes. In theory, the focus of treatment in such facilities is to prepare the child for a return to a foster home, to an adoptive home, or to the birth parents when applicable. But two major reviews of the scholarly literature have questioned these facilities' effectiveness.[7] There are some children in foster care who are difficult to place in permanent homes through the normal adoption process. These children are often said to require "special-needs adoption." In this context, "special needs" can include situations where children have specific chronic medical problems, mental health issues, behavioral problems, and learning disabilities. In some cases, sibling groups, and older children qualify as "special needs."[8] Governments offer a variety of incentives and services to facilitate this class of adoptions.[9]

Funding and system incentives

A law passed by Congress in 1961 allowed AFDC (welfare) payments to pay for foster care which was previously made only to children in their own homes. This made aided funding foster care for states and localities, facilitating rapid growth. In some cases, the state of Texas paid mental treatment centers as much as $101,105 a year per child. Observers of the growth trend note that a county will only continue to receive funding while it keeps the child in its care. This may create a "perverse financial incentive" to place and retain children in foster care rather than leave them with their parents, and incentives are sometimes set up for maximum intervention. A National Coalition for Child Protection Reform issue paper states "children often are removed from their families `prematurely or unnecessarily' because federal aid formulas give states `a strong financial incentive' to do so rather than provide services to keep families together."[10]

Findings of a grand jury investigation in Santa Clara, California:[11]

> The Grand Jury heard from staff members of the DFCS and others outside the department that the department puts too much money into "back-end services," i.e., therapists and attorneys, and not enough money into "front-end" or basic services. The county does not receive as much in federal funds for "front-end" services, which could help solve the problems causing family inadequacies, as it receives for out-of-home placements or foster care services. In other words, the Agency benefits, financially, from placing children in foster homes.

United States

Foster care legislation since 1990

In 1997, the Adoption and Safe Families Act (ASFA) was passed.[12] This reduced the time children are allowed to remain in foster care before being available for adoption. The new law requires state child welfare agencies to identify cases where "aggravated circumstances" make permanent separation of child from the birth family the best option for the safety and well-being of the child. One of the main components of ASFA is the imposition of stricter time limits on reunification efforts. Proponents of ASFA claimed that before the law was passed, the lack of such legislation was the reason it was common for children to languish in care for years with no permanent living situation identified.

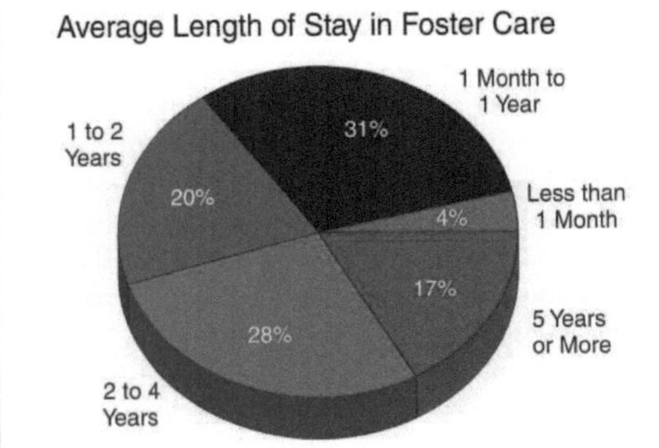

Source: Adoption and Foster Care Analysis and Reporting System, interim FY 2000 data.

Average length of stay in foster care in the U.S.

Opponents of ASFA argued that the real reason children languished in foster care was that too many were taken needlessly from their parents in the first place. Since ASFA did not address this, opponents said, it would not accomplish its goals, and would only slow a decline in the foster care population that should have occurred anyway because of a decline in reported child abuse.[13]

Ten years after ASFA became law, the number of children in foster care on any given day has been about 7,000 fewer than when ASFA was passed[14]

The Foster Care Independence Act of 1999, helps foster youth who are aging out of care to achieve self-sufficiency. The U.S. government has also funded the Education and Training Voucher Program in recent years in order to help youth who age out of care to obtain college or vocational training at a free or reduced cost. Chafee and ETV money is administered by each state as they see fit.

The Fostering Connections to Success and Increasing Adoptions Act of 2008 is the most recent piece of major federal legislation addressing the foster care system. This bill extended various benefits and funding for foster children between the age of 18 and 21 and for Indian children in tribal areas. The legislation also strengthens requirements for states in their treatment of siblings and introduces mechanisms to provide financial incentives for guardianship and adoption.[15] [16]

Constitutional issues

In May 2007, the United States 9th Circuit Court of Appeals found in ROGERS v. COUNTY OF SAN JOAQUIN, No. 05-16071[17] that a CPS social worker who removed children from their natural parents into foster care without obtaining judicial authorization, was acting without due process and without exigency (emergency conditions) violated the 14th Amendment and Title 42 United State Code Section 1983. The Fourteenth Amendment to the United States Constitution says that a state may not make a law that abridges "... the privileges or immunities of citizens of the United States" and no state may "deprive any person of life, liberty, or property, without due process of law; nor deny to any person within its jurisdiction the equal protection of the laws." Title 42 United States Code Section 1983[18] states that citizens can sue in federal courts any person that acting under a color of law to deprive the citizens of their civil rights under the pretext of a regulation of a state.[19]

In case of Santosky v. Kramer, 455 US 745, Supreme Court reviewed a case when Department of Social Services removed two younger children from their natural parents only because the parents had been previously found negligent toward their oldest daughter.[20] When the third child was only three days old, DSS transferred him to a foster home on the ground that immediate removal was necessary to avoid imminent danger to his life or health. The Supreme Court vacated previous judgment and stated: "Before a State may sever completely and irrevocably the rights of parents in their natural child, due process requires that the State support its allegations by at least clear and convincing evidence. <..> But until the State proves parental unfitness, the child and his parents share a vital interest in preventing erroneous termination of their natural relationship".[20]

Also District of Columbia Court of Appeals conclude that the lower trial court erred in rejecting the relative custodial arrangement selected by the natural mother who tried to preserve her relationship with the child.[21] The previous judgment granting the foster mother's adoption petition was reversed, and the case remanded to the trial court to vacate the orders granting adoption and denying custody, and to enter an order granting custody to the child's relative.[21]

In 2007 Deanna Fogarty-Hardwick obtained a jury verdict against Orange County (California) and two of its social workers for violating her Fourteenth Amendment rights to familial association by unlawfully placing her kids in foster care.[22] The $4.9 million verdict grew to a $9.5 million judgment as the County lost each of its successive appeals.[22] The case finally ended in 2011 when the United States Supreme Court denied Orange County's request to overturn the verdict.[23]

Australia

Home-based care, which includes foster care, is provided to children who are in need of care and protection. Children and young people are provided with alternative accommodation while they are unable to live with their parents. As well as foster care, this can include placements with relatives or kin, and residential care. In most cases, children in home-based care are also on a care and protection order.[24]

In some cases children are placed in home-based care following a child protection substantiation and where they are found to be in need of a safer and more stable environment. In other situations parents may be incapable of providing adequate care for the child, or accommodation may be needed during times of family conflict or crisis.[24] In the significant number of cases substance abuse is a major contributing factor.

Respite care is a type of foster care that is used to provide short-term (and often regular) accommodation for children whose parents are ill or unable to care for them on a temporary basis.[24] It is also used to provide a break for the parent or primary carer to hopefully decrease the chances of the situation escalating to one which would lead to the removal of the child(ren).

As with the majority of child protection services, states and territories are responsible for funding home-based care. Non-government organizations are widely used, however, to provide these services.[24]

The Lost Children (Britain-Australia)

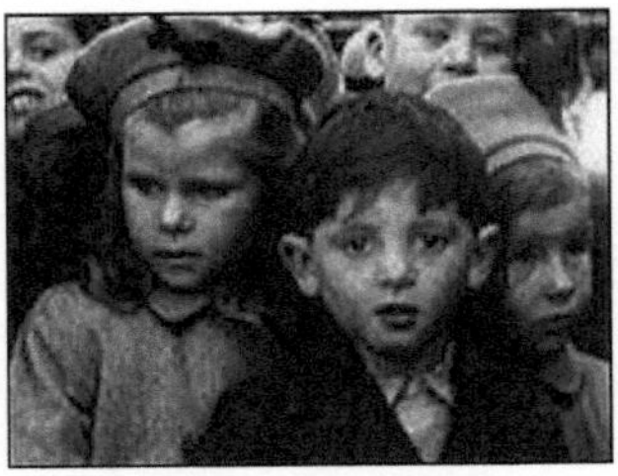
Children of the United Kingdom's Children's Migrant Programme

An estimated 150,000 British children were sent to overseas colonies and countries in the commonwealth such as Australia. This practice was in effect from the beginning of the nineteenth century until 1967. Many of these children were sent to orphanages, foster homes and religious institutions, where they were used as a free source of labour and many were severely abused and neglected. These children were classified as orphans although most were not. In the period after World War II the policy was dubbed the "Child Migrants Programme". The prime consideration was money as it was cheaper to care for children in commonwealth countries than it was in the United Kingdom. At least 10,000 children, some as young as 3, were shipped to Australia after the war,[25] [26] most to join the ranks of the "Forgotten Australians", the term given for those who experienced care in foster homes and institutions in the 20th century. Among these Forgotten Australians were members of the "Stolen Generation", the children of Australian Aborigines, forcibly removed from their homes and raised in white institutions. In 2008 Australian Prime Minister, Kevin Rudd apologised to the approximately 500,000 "forgotten Australians" and in 2010 British Prime Minister Gordon Brown issued a similar apology to those who were victimised by the Child Migrants Programme.[27] [28] [29]

Current policy

There is strong emphasis in current Australian policy and practice to keep children with their families wherever possible. In the event that children are placed in home-based care, every effort is made to reunite children with their families wherever possible.[24]

In the case of Aboriginal and Torres Strait Islander children in particular, but not exclusively, placing the child within the wider family or community is preferred[24] This is consistent with the Aboriginal Child Placement Principle.[30]

Negative effects

Individuals who were in foster care experience higher rates of physical and psychiatric morbidity than the general population and suffer from not being able to trust and that can lead to placements breaking down.[31] In a study of adults who were in foster care in Oregon and Washington state, they were found to have double the incidence of depression, 20% as compared to 10% and were found to have a higher rate of post-traumatic stress disorder (PTSD) than combat veterans with 25% of those studied having PTSD. Children in foster care have a higher probability of having Attention Deficit Hyperactivity Disorder, and deficits in executive functioning, anxiety as well as other developmental problems.[32] [33] [34] [35] These children experience higher degrees of incarceration, poverty, homelessness, and suicide. Recent studies in the U.S. suggest that foster care placements are more detrimental to children than remaining in a troubled home.[36] [37] [38]

Neurodevelopment

Foster care has been shown in various studies to have deleterious consequences on the physical health and mental wellbeing of those who were in foster care. Many children enter foster care at a very young age, a period where the development of mental and psychological processes are at one of their critical peaks. The human brain doesn't fully develop until approximately the age of 25,[39] and one of the most critical periods of brain development occurs in the first 3–4 years. The processes that govern the development of personality traits, stress response and cognitive skills are formed during this period. The developing brain is directly influenced by negative environmental factors including lack of stimulation due to emotional neglect, poor nutrition, exposure to violence in the home environment and child abuse.

Negative environmental influences have a direct effect on all areas of neurodevelopment: neurogenesis (creation of new neurons), apoptosis (death and reabsorption of neurons), migration (of neurons to different regions of the brain), synaptogenesis (creation of synapses), synaptic sculpturing (determining the make-up of the synapse), arborization (the growth of dendritic connections, myelinzation (protective covering of neurons), and an enlargement of the brain's ventricles, which can cause cortical atrophy.

Most of the processes involved in healthy neurodevelopment are predicated upon the establishment of close nurturing relationships and environmental stimulation. Foster children have elevated levels of cortisol, a stress hormone in comparison to children raised by their biological parents. Elevated cortisol levels can compromise the immune system. (Harden BJ, 2004).[40] Negative environmental influences during this critical period of brain development can have lifelong consequences.[41] [42] [43] [44]

Epigenetic effects of environment

Gene expression can be affected by the environment through epigenetic mechanisms. Negative environmental influences, such as maternal deprivation, child abuse and stress[45] [46] have been shown to have a profound effect on gene expression, including transgenerational epigenetic effects in which physiological and behavioral (intellectual) transfer of information across generations-not-yet-conceived is effected. In the Överkalix study in Sweden, the effects of epigentic inheritance were shown to have a direct correlation to the environmental influences faced by the parents and grandparents.[47] Many physiological and behavioral characteristics ascribed to Mendelian inheritance are due in fact to transgenerational epigenetic inheritance. The implications in terms of foster care and the cost to society as a whole is that the stress, deprivation and other negative environmental factors many foster children are subjected to has a detrimental effect not only their physical, emotional and cognitive well-being, but that the damage can transcend generations.[48] [49] [50]

In studies of the adult offspring of Holocaust survivors, parental PTSD was a risk factor for the development of PTSD in adult offspring in comparison to those whose parents went through the Holocaust without developing PTSD. The offspring of survivors with PTSD had lower levels of urinary cortisol excretion, salivary cortisol and enhanced plasma cortisol suppression in response to low dose dexamethasone administration than offspring of survivors without PTSD. Low cortisol levels are associated with parental, particularly maternal, PTSD. This is in contrast to the normal stress response in which cortisol levels are elevated after exposure to a stressor. The results of the study point to the involvement of epigenetic mechanisms.[51] [52]

Epigenetic Effects of Abuse
"In addition, the effects of abuse may extend beyond the immediate victim into subsequent generations as a consequence of epigenetic effects transmitted directly to offspring and/or behavioral changes in affected individuals. (Neighh GN *et al.* 2009)[53]

It has been suggested in various studies that the deleterious epigentic effects may be somewhat ameliorated through pharmacological manipulations in adulthood via the administration of nerve growth factor-inducible protein A,[54] and through the inhibition of a class of enzymes known as the histone deacetylases (HDACs). *"HDAC inhibitors (HDACIs) such as Trichostatin A (TSA);* "TSA can be used to alter gene expression by interfering with the removal of acetyl groups from histones", *and L-methionine an essential amino acid, have been developed for the treatment of a variety of malignancies and neurodegenerative disorders. Drug combination approaches have also shown promise for the treatment of mood disorders including bipolar disorder, anxiety and depression."*[55] [56]

Post traumatic stress disorder

Children in foster care have a higher incidence of Post traumatic stress disorder (PTSD).In one study (Dubner and Motta, 1999)[58] 60% of children in foster care who had experienced sexual abuse had PTSD, and 42% of those who had been physically abused fulfilled the PTSD criteria. PTSD was also found in 18% of the children who were not abused. These children may have developed PTSD due to witnessing violence in the home. (Marsenich, 2002).

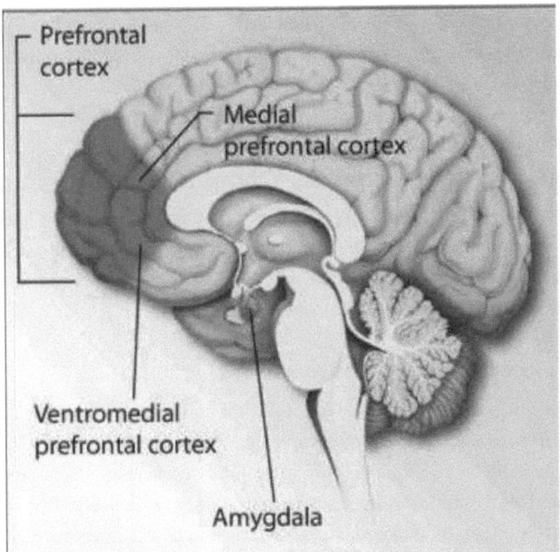

Regions of the brain associated with stress and post traumatic stress disorder[57]

In a study conducted in Oregon and Washington state, the rate of PTSD in adults who were in foster care for one year between the ages of 14–18 was found to be higher than that of combat veterans, with 25 percent of those in the study meeting the diagnostic criteria as compared to 12–13 percent of Iraq war veterans and 15 percent of Vietnam war veterans, and a rate of 4% in the general population. The recovery rate for foster home alumni was 28.2% as opposed to 47% in the general population.

"More than half the study participants reported clinical levels of mental illness, compared to less than a quarter of the general population".[59] [60]

Eating disorders

Foster children are at increased risk for a variety of eating disorders, in comparison to the general population.

Obesity: Children in foster care are more prone to becoming overweight and obese, and in a study done in the United Kingdom, 35% of foster children experienced an increase in Body Mass Index (BMI) once in care.[61]

Hyperphagic Short Stature syndrome (HSS) is a condition characterized by short stature due to insufficient growth hormone production, an excessive appetite (hyperphagia) and mild learning disabilities. While it is believed to have genetic component, HSS is triggered by being exposed to an environment of high psychosocial stress; it is not uncommon in children in foster homes or other stressful environments. HSS improves upon removal from the stressful environment.[62] [63] [64]

Food Maintenance Syndrome is characterized by a set of aberrant eating behaviors of children in foster care. It is "a pattern of excessive eating and food acquisition and maintenance behaviors without concurrent obesity"; it resembles "the behavioral correlates of Hyperphagic Short Stature". It is hypothesised that this syndrome is triggered by the stress and maltreatment foster children are subjected to, it was prevalent amongst 25 percent of the study group in New Zealand.[33]

Bulimia Nervosa is seven times more prevalent among former foster children than in the general population.[65]

Disorganized attachment

A study by Dante Cicchetti found that 80% of abused and maltreated infants in his study exhibited symptoms of disorganized attachment.[66] [67] Children with histories of maltreatment, such as physical and psychological neglect, physical abuse, and sexual abuse, are at risk of developing psychiatric problems.[68] [69] [70] [71] These children may be described as experiencing trauma as the result of abuse or neglect, inflicted by a primary caregiver, which disrupts the normal development of secure attachment. Such children are at risk of developing a disorganized attachment.[70] [72] [73] Disorganized attachment is associated with a number of developmental problems, including dissociative symptoms,[74] as well as depressive, anxiety, and acting-out symptoms.[75] [76]

Poverty and homelessness

Nearly half of foster kids in the U.S. become homeless when they turn 18.[77] [78] "One of every 10 foster children stays in foster care longer than seven years, and each year about 15,000 reach the age of majority and leave foster care without a permanent family—many to join the ranks of the homeless or to commit crimes and be imprisoned.[79] [80]

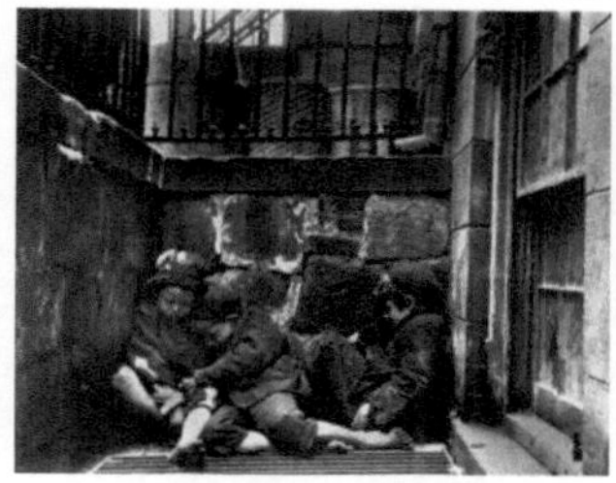

New York street children; 1890

Three out of 10 of the United States homeless are former foster children.[81] According to the results of the Casey Family Study of Foster Care Alumni, up to 80 percent are doing poorly—with a quarter to a third of former foster children at or below the poverty line, three times the national poverty rate.[82] Very frequently, people who are homeless had multiple placements as children: some were in foster care, but others experienced "unofficial" placements in the homes of family or friends.

Individuals with a history foster care tend to become homeless at an earlier age than those who were not in foster care . The length of time a person remains homeless is prolonged in indiviuals who were in foster care.[83]

Suicide-death rate

Children in foster care are at a greater risk of suicide,[84] the increased risk of suicide is still prevalent after leaving foster care and occurs at a higher rate than the general population. In a small study of twenty-two Texan youths who aged out of the system, 23 percent had a history of suicide attempts.[85]

A Swedish study utilizing the data of almost one million people including 22,305 former foster children who had been in care prior to their teens, concluded:

> Former child welfare clients were in year of birth and sex standardised risk ratios (RRs) four to five times more likely than peers in the general population to have been hospitalised for suicide attempts....Individuals who had been in long-term foster care tended to have the most dismal outcome...former child welfare/protection clients should be considered a high-risk group for suicide attempts and severe psychiatric morbidity.[86]

Death rate

Children in foster care have an overall higher mortality rate than children in the general population.[87] A study conducted in Finland among current and former foster children up to age 24 found a higher mortality rate due to substance abuse, accidents, suicide and illness. The deaths due to illness were attributed to an increased incidence of acute and chronic medical conditions and developmental delays among children in foster care.[88]

Georgia Senator Nancy Schaefer published a report "The Corrupt Business of Child Protective Services"[89] stating:

> "The National Center on Child Abuse and Neglect in 1998 reported that six times as many children died in foster care than in the general public and that once removed to official “safety”, these children are far

more likely to suffer abuse, including sexual molestation than in the general population".[89]

Poor academic prospects

Educational outcomes of ex-foster children in the Northwest Alumni Study*[90]
• 56% completed high school compared to 82% of the general population, although an additional 29% of former foster children received a G.E.D. compared to an additional 5% of the general population. • 42.7% completed some education beyond high school. • 20.6% completed any degree or certificate beyond high school • 16.1% completed a vocational degree; 21.9% for those over 25. • 1.8% complete a bachelors degree, 2.7% for over 25, the completion rate for the general population in the same age group is 24%, a sizable difference.
*The study reviewed case records for 659 foster care alumni in Northwest USA, and interviewed 479 of them between September 2000 and January 2002.[90]

Several studies have indicated that foster care children tend to underachieve academically with many never completing high school. In a study conducted in Philadelphia by Johns Hopkins University it was found that; among high school students who are in foster care, have been abused and neglected, or receive out of home placement by the courts, the probability of dropping out of school is greater than 75%.[91]

State abuses

Drug testing

Throughout the 1990s, experimental HIV drugs were tested on HIV-positive foster children at Incarnation Children's Center in Harlem. The agency has also been accused of racism, some comparing the trials to the Tuskegee syphilis experiment, as 98 percent of children in foster care in New York City belong to ethnic minorities.[92]

Unnecessary/over medication

Studies[93] have revealed that youth in foster care covered by Medicaid insurance receive psychotropic medication at a rate that was 3 times higher than that of Medicaid-insured youth who qualify by low family income. In a review (September 2003 to August 2004) of the medical records of 32,135 Texas foster care 0–19 years-old, 12,189 were prescribed psychotropic medication, resulting in an annual prevalence of 37.9% of these children being prescribed medication. 41.3% received 3 different classes of these drugs during July 2004, and 15.9% received 4 different classes. The most frequently used medications were antidepressants (56.8%), attention-deficit/hyperactivity disorder drugs (55.9%), and antipsychotic agents (53.2%).

> "Concomitant psychotropic medication treatment is frequent for youth in foster care and lacks substantive evidence as to its effectiveness and safety".[93]
>
> — Psychotropic medication patterns among youth in foster care., *Pediatrics 2008*

Psychiatrists prescribed 93% of the psychotropic medication, and it was noted in the review of these cases that the use of expensive, brand name, patent protected medication was prevalent. In the case of SSRIs the use of the most expensive medications was noted to be 74%, in the general market only 28% are for brand name SSRI's vs generics. The average out-of-pocket expense per prescription was $34.75 for generics and $90.17 for branded products, a $55.42, difference.[94]

Abuse and negligence

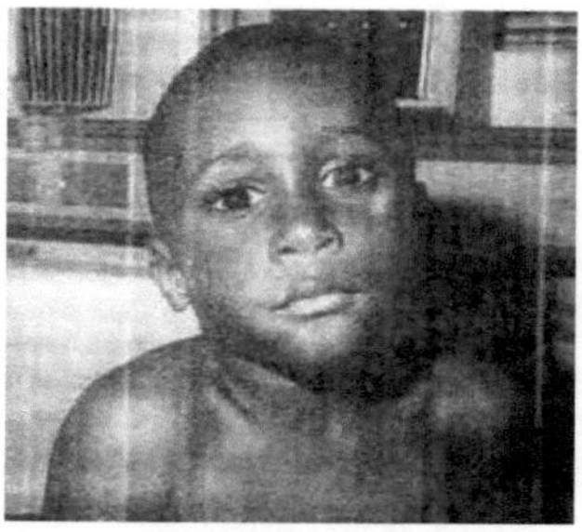

Only known photograph of five-year-old Georgia resident Terrell Peterson while alive, taken shortly before his murder at the hands of his foster parent. The case was covered up by the Georgia Department of Children and Family Services.

Children in foster care experience high rates of child abuse, emotional deprivation, and physical neglect. In one study in the United Kingdom "foster children were 7–8 times, and children in residential care 6 times more likely to be assessed by a pediatrician for abuse than a child in the general population".[95] One study by Johns Hopkins University found that the rate of sexual abuse within the foster-care system is more than four times as high as in the general population; in group homes, the rate of sexual abuse is more than 28 times that of the general population.[96] [97] An Indiana study found three times more physical abuse and twice the rate of sexual abuse in foster homes than in the general population [97] A study of foster children in Oregon and Washington State found that nearly one third reported being abused by a foster parent or another adult in a foster home.[98] These statistics do not speak to the situation these children are coming from, but it does show the very large problem of child-on-child sexual abuse within the system. There have been several notable lawsits concerning sexual abuse and negligence that caused review of the foster care system in some states:

In 2010, an ex-foster child was awarded $30 million by jury trial in California (Santa Clara County) for sexual abuse damages that happened to him in his foster home from 1995 to 1999.[99] [100] The foster parent, John Jackson, was licensed by the state, despite the fact that he abused his own wife and son, overdosed on drugs and was arrested for drunken driving. In 2006 Jackson was convicted in Santa Clara County of nine counts of lewd or lascivious acts on a child by force, violence, duress, menace and fear, and seven counts of lewd or lascivious acts on a child under 14, according to the Santa Clara County District Attorney's Office.[99] The sex acts that he forced the children in his foster care to perform sent him to prison for 220 years. Later in 2010, Giarretto Institute, the private foster family agency responsible for licensing and monitoring Jackson's foster home and others, was also found to be negligent and liable for 75 percent of the abuse that was inflicted on the victim, and Jackson himself was liable for the rest.[99]

In 2009, Oregon Department of Human Services agreed to pay $2 million into a fund for the future care of twins who were allegedly abused by their foster parents; this was the largest such settlement in the agency's history.[101] According to the civil rights suit filed on request of the twins' adoptive mother in December 2007 in U.S. Federal Court, the children were kept in makeshift cages—cribs covered with chicken wire secured by duct tape—in a darkened bedroom known as "the dungeon." The brother and sister often went without food, water or human touch. The boy, who had a shunt put into his head at birth to drain fluid, did not receive medical attention, so when police rescued the twins he was nearly comatose. The same foster family previously took into their care hundreds of other children over nearly four decades.[102] DHS said the foster parents deceived child welfare workers during the checkup visits.[101]

Several lawsuits were brought in 2008 against the Florida Department of Children & Families (DCF), accusing it of mishandling reports that Thomas Ferrara, 79, a foster parent, was molesting young girls.[103] [104] The suits claimed that even though there were records of sexual misconduct allegations against Ferrara in 1992, 1996, and 1999, the DCF continued to place foster children with Ferrara and his then-wife until 2000.[103] Ferrara was arrested in 2001, after a 9-year-old girl told detectives he regularly molested her over two years and threatened to hurt her mother if she told anyone. Records show that Ferrara had as many as 400 children go through his home during his 16 years as a licensed foster parent (from 1984 to 2000).[103] Officials stated that the lawsuits over Ferrara ended up costing the DCF almost $2.26 million.[104] Similarly, in 2007 Florida's DCF paid $1.2 million to settle a lawsuit that alleged DCF ignored complaints that another mentally disabled Immokalee girl was being raped by her foster father,

Bonifacio Velazquez, until the 15-year-old gave birth to a child.[105] [106] [107]

In a class action lawsuit Charlie and Nadine H. v. McGreevey[108] was filed in federal court by "Children's Rights" New York organization on behalf of children in the custody of the New Jersey Division of Youth and Family Services (DYFS).[109] [110] The complaint alleged violations of the childrens' constitutional rights and their rights under Title IV-E of the Social Security Act, the Child Abuse Prevention and Treatment Act, Early Periodic Screening Diagnosis and Treatment, 504 of the Rehabilitation Act, the Americans with Disabilities Act, and the Multiethnic Placement Act (MEPA).[111] In July 2002, the federal court granted plaintiffs' experts access to 500 children's case files, allowing plaintiffs to collect information concerning harm to children in foster care through a case record review.[109] These files revealed numerous cases in which foster children were abused, and DYFS failed to take proper action. On June 9, 2004, the child welfare panel appointed by the parties approved the NJ State's Reform Plan. The court accepted the plan on June 17, 2004.[110] The same organization also filed similar lawsuits against several other states in recent years that caused some of the states to start child welfare reforms.[112]

In the United Kingdom a convicted pedophile was allowed to become a foster parent despite having served three years in prison for sexually abusing a Boy Scout. The convicted pedophile – David Mason – was allowed to have a foster child placed with him because the Kent County Council did not have his identity checked. Mason is currently incarcerated for numerous charges including rape.[113]

In Nottinghamshire County in the UK an ex-foster father was convicted in 2010 of raping and sexually abusing vulnerable boys for more than a decade.[114]

Strip Searches

Sometimes children who have been taken from their homes due to abuse or neglect are temporarily placed into shelters if a foster home is not immediately available. Some of these shelters are wings of juvenile detention facilities. Sometimes the foster children placed into these shelter wings are subjected to strip searches similar to those performed on juvenile offenders.[115]

Therapeutic intervention

The negative physical, psychological, cognitive and epigenetic effects of foster care have been established in innumerable studies in various countries. The Casey Family Programs Northwest Foster Care Alumni Study was a fairly extensive study into various aspects of the psychosocial effects of foster care noted that 80% of ex-foster children are doing "poorly".

Neuroplasticity

The human brain however has been shown to have a fair degree of neuroplasticity.[116] [117] [118] Adult neurogenesis has been shown to be an ongoing process.[119]

"... all those experiences are of much significance which show how the judgment of the senses may be modified by experience and by training derived under various circumstances, and may be adapted to the new conditions..." – Hermann von Helmholtz, 1866

While having a background in foster homes—especially in instances of sexual abuse—can be the precipitating factor in a wide variety of psychological and cognitive deficits such as ADHD,[120] and PTSD,[58] [121] it may also serve to obfuscate the true cause of underlying issues. The foster care experience may have nothing to do with the symptoms, or on the other hand, the symptoms may be exacerbated by having a history of foster care and the attendant abuses.

Children in the child welfare system have often experienced significant and repeated traumas. Dyadic Developmental Psychotherapy is one of the approaches that has been used to treat the resulting trauma and attachment difficulties caused by chronic early maltreatment within a care-giving relationship.[122] [123] [124]

Foster Parent and Child Reunions

Foster parents play an important pivotal role in the lives of infants placed in their care during critical developmental periods. When orphaned, fostered, or adopted children suffering from genealogical bewilderment are curious to learn about their family background and medial history, searches to locate former foster parents have potential to be just as captivating, technically challenging, and convoluted as searching for biological parents. A successful reunion with a loving set of benevolent caregiving foster parents also has potential to create positive emotional responses, stimulate happiness through an increased sense of connectedness and sense of indebtedness for children who were fostered.[125]

Foster care in popular culture

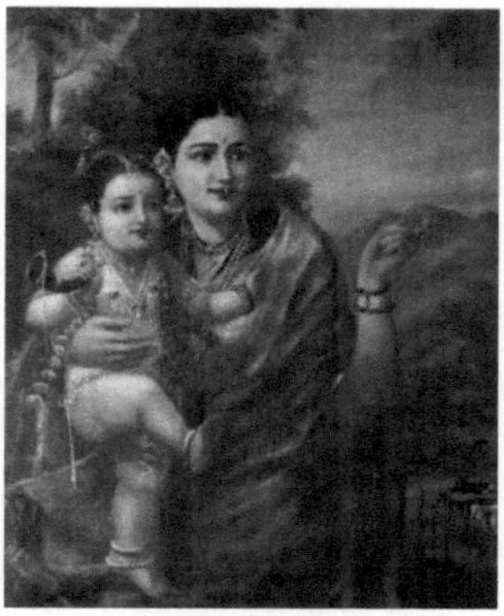

Raja Ravi Varma's Painting of Sri Krishna, as a young child with foster mother Yasoda

- Fictional characters
  - In the Fox television show *Bones*, forensic anthropologist Dr. Temperance Brennan (played by Emily Deschanel) grew up in foster care when her parents went missing. Dr. Sweets was also in foster care until he got adopted at six.[126]
  - ABC's *Secret Life of the American Teenager*'s Ricky (played by Dareen Kagasoff) is in foster care.[127]
  - On TNT's *Leverage*, Parker (played by Beth Riesgraf) and Hardison (played by Aldis Hodge) both grew up in foster care. While Hardison had a good experience with his "nana", Parker had several bad experiences with several bad foster families.[128][129]
  - The main and title character in the book *The Great Gilly Hopkins* is a foster child who wishes to be reunited with their mother.
  - The main characters in the film *Money Train* were foster brothers of different races (played by Wesley Snipes and Woody Harrelson).
  - Sean Kennedy and Emma Kennedy BBC *Hustle (TV series)* Sean and Emma were put into foster care after their mother died .
  - The main character, Lux, in *Life Unexpected (TV series)* played by Brittney Robertson grew up in foster care and later sought out her parents to gain emancipation from the foster care system. When failing, she is later adopted by her biological parents.
  - The main and title character in the childrens book *The Story of Tracy Beaker* by Jacqueline Wilson, Tracy is put into foster care as a result of neglect.
  - The main character in the ABC Family Television show ' ' The Lying Game ' ', Emma Becker, grew up in foster care while her twin sister Sutton Mercer grew up in a privileged adopted family.
- Famous former foster children
  - Allison Anders, writer and director
  - Alonzo Mourning, NBA Defensive Player of the Year in 1999 & 2000 and seven-time NBA All-Star
  - Babe Ruth, American Major League baseball player
  - Eddie Murphy, actor
  - Eriq La Salle, actor
  - Esai Morales, actor
  - Marilyn Monroe, actress, singer and model
  - Victoria Rowell, dancer[130]

- Wayne Dyer, author and motivational speaker
- Leland Chapman, Son of Duane Dog Chapman

See also

- Attachment theory
- Complex post-traumatic stress disorder
- Crown ward
- Foster care adoption
- Grandfamily
- Reactive attachment disorder
- Residential education

References

[1] Dorsey et Al. *Current status and evidence base of training for foster and treatment foster parents*

[2] "Pew Commission on Children in Foster Care "Demographics of Children in Foster Care"" (http://pewfostercare.org/research/docs/Demographics0903.pdf). Pewfostercare.org. . Retrieved 2011-11-01.

[3] "Fewer U.S. kids in foster care" (http://www.google.com/hostednews/ap/article/ALeqM5gq1yhAPK8txoVpGAPujSMUK9wz5gD9HULPCG4). Burlington, Vermont: Burlington Free Press. 1 September 2010. pp. 1A. .

[4] "About Foster Children" (http://www.adoptuskids.org/resourceCenter/about-children-in-foster-care.aspx). Adoptuskids.org. . Retrieved 2011-11-01.

[5] "Pew Commission on Children in Foster Care" (http://pewfostercare.org/). Pewfostercare.org. . Retrieved 2011-11-01.

[6] "Children's Bureau Website – Child Welfare Monitoring" (http://www.acf.hhs.gov/programs/cb/cwmonitoring/index.htm). Acf.hhs.gov. . Retrieved 2011-11-01.

[7] Richard Barth, *Institutions vs. Foster Homes, the Empirical Base for a Century of Action* (University of North Carolina, Jordan Institute for Families, February 17, 2002; U.S. Department of Health and Human Services, *Report of the Surgeon General's Conference on children's mental health: A national action agenda.* Washington, D.C: Government Printing Office, 2000.USGPO

[8] "Common Myths About Adoption" (http://www.adoptuskids.org/resourceCenter/specialNeeds.aspx). AdoptUSKids. . Retrieved 2011-11-01.

[9] JSTOR (http://www.jstor.org/pss/1602402), Judith K. McKenzie. Adoption of Children with Special Needs, Brookings Institution: The Future of Children, Vol. 3, No. 1, Adoption (Spring, 1993), pp. 62–76

[10] Child Abuse is Child Protection is Mental Health Treatment is Drugging Children (http://www.wildestcolts.com/safeEducation/cps.html)

[11] 1992–93 Santa Clara County Grand Jury, Final Report, Investigation: Department Of Family And Children's Services, 1993.

[12] Children's Bureau Express Online Digest: (http://cbexpress.acf.hhs.gov/nonissart.cfm?issue_id=2006-09&disp_art=1221)

[13] U.S. Dept. of Health and Human Services, *Child Maltreatment, 2004*, Figure 3-2, HHS.gov (http://www.acf.hhs.gov/programs/cb/pubs/cm04/figure3_2.htm)

[14] As of March, 1998, four months after ASFA became law, there were 520,000 children in foster care, (U.S. Department of Health and Human Services, *AFCARS Report #1*. HHS.gov (http://www.acf.hhs.gov/programs/cb/stats_research/afcars/tar/report1/ar0199.htm) It took until September 30, 2005, for the number to fall to 513,000 (U.S. Department of Health and Human Services, *Trends in Foster Care and Adoption*, HHS.gov (http://www.acf.hhs.gov/programs/cb/stats_research/afcars/trends.htm)

[15] "Fostering Connections to Success and Increasing Adoptions Act" (http://www.childrensdefense.org/helping-americas-children/child-welfare/fostering-connection-success-increasing-adoptions-act-overview.html). Childrensdefense.org. 2008-10-07. . Retrieved 2011-11-01.

[16] (http://www.ncsl.org/statefed/humserv/SummaryHR6893.htm)

[17] "ROGERS v. COUNTY OF SAN JOAQUIN, No. 05-16071" (http://caselaw.findlaw.com/us-9th-circuit/1083074.html). Caselaw.findlaw.com. . Retrieved 2011-11-01.

[18] "Title 42 United States Code Section 1983" (http://www.law.cornell.edu/uscode/42/usc_sec_42_00001983----000-.html). Law.cornell.edu. 2010-10-15. . Retrieved 2011-11-01.

[19] "Civil Rights Complaint Guide" (http://www.utd.uscourts.gov/forms/civilrt_guide.pdf). .

[20] "Santosky v. Kramer, 455 US 745 – Supreme Court 1982" (http://scholar.google.com/scholar_case?case=16163171324148079216). .

[21] "In re TJ, 666 A. 2d 1 – DC: Court of Appeals 1995" (http://scholar.google.com/scholar_case?case=3149611456727370759&hl). .

[22] "Order Granting Fees Incurred on Appeal" (http://www.jdsupra.com/post/documentViewer.aspx?fid=6cdf672e-9fc7-4ab4-a5a8-8d1372e3c918). .

[23] "U.S. Supreme Court Denies Orange County's (California) Request" (http://www.prweb.com/releases/2011FogartyHardwick/04CertDenied/prweb5261414.htm). .

[24] "Child protection Australia 2005–06 (full publication; 19/12/2007 edition) (AIHW)" (http://www.aihw.gov.au/publications/cws/cpa05-06/cpa05-06.pdf) (PDF). . Retrieved 2011-11-01.

[25] "The Lost Children" (http://www.cbsnews.com/stories/1999/03/24/60II/main40269.shtml). Cbsnews.com. 2009-02-11. . Retrieved 2011-11-01.

[26] "Lost childhood of Laurie Humphreys, British migrant sent to Australia" (http://www.timesonline.co.uk/tol/news/world/article6918770.ece?token=null&offset=0&page=1). Timesonline.co.uk. 2011-02-15. . Retrieved 2011-11-01.

[27] "British Child Migration to Australia: History, Senate Inquiry and Responsibilities" (http://www.murdoch.edu.au/elaw/issues/v9n4/buti94.html). Murdoch.edu.au. . Retrieved 2011-11-01.

[28] "Australia 'sorry' for child abuse" (http://news.bbc.co.uk/2/hi/8361389.stm). BBC News. 2009-11-16. . Retrieved 2011-11-01.

[29] "Gordon Brown apologises to British children who were abused after being sent abroad to start better life" (http://www.dailyrecord.co.uk/news/uk-world-news/2010/02/24/gordon-brown-apologises-for-programme-which-saw-thousands-of-british-children-to-colonies-to-be-abused-86908-22066649/). Dailyrecord.co.uk. . Retrieved 2011-11-01.

[30] "Research Report 7 (1997) – The Aboriginal Child Placement Principle" (http://www.lawlink.nsw.gov.au/lrc.nsf/pages/RR7TOC). Lawlink NSW. 2001-06-05. . Retrieved 2011-11-01.

[31] McCann, JB; James, A; Wilson, S; Dunn, G (1996). "Prevalence of psychiatric disorders in young people in the care system". *BMJ (Clinical research ed.)* **313** (7071): 1529–30. PMC 2353045. PMID 8978231.

[32] Pears, K; Fisher, PA (2005). "Developmental, cognitive, and neuropsychological functioning in preschool-aged foster children: associations with prior maltreatment and placement history". *Journal of developmental and behavioral pediatrics : JDBP* **26** (2): 112–22. PMID 15827462.

[33] Tarren-Sweeney, M; Hazell, P (2006). "Mental health of children in foster and kinship care in New South Wales, Australia". *Journal of paediatrics and child health* **42** (3): 89–97. doi:10.1111/j.1440-1754.2006.00804.x. PMID 16509906.

[34] Pecora, PJ; Jensen, PS; Romanelli, LH; Jackson, LJ; Ortiz, A (2009). "Mental health services for children placed in foster care: an overview of current challenges". *Child welfare* **88** (1): 5–26. PMC 3061347. PMID 19653451.

[35] Karnik, Niranjan S. (2000). *Journal of Medical Humanities* **21** (4): 199. doi:10.1023/A:1009073008365.

[36] "Child Protection and Child Outcomes: Measuring the Effects of Foster Care" (http://www.mit.edu/~jjdoyle/doyle_fosterlt_march07_aer.pdf) (PDF). . Retrieved 2011-11-01.

[37] Koch, Wendy (2007-07-03). "Study: Troubled homes better than foster care" (http://www.usatoday.com/news/nation/2007-07-02-foster-study_N.htm). Usatoday.Com. . Retrieved 2011-11-01.

[38] Lawrence, CR; Carlson, EA; Egeland, B (2006). "The impact of foster care on development". *Development and psychopathology* **18** (1): 57–76. doi:10.1017/S0954579406060044. PMID 16478552.

[39] http://www.academic.marist.edu/mwwatch/fall05/science1.htm

[40] Harden, BJ (2004). "Safety and stability for foster children: a developmental perspective". *The Future of children / Center for the Future of Children, the David and Lucile Packard Foundation* **14** (1): 30–47. PMID 15072017.

[41] "American Academy of Pediatrics. Committee on Early Childhood and Adoption and Dependent Care. Developmental issues for young children in foster care". *Pediatrics* **106** (5): 1145–50. 2000. PMID 11061791.

[42] Silverman, AB; Reinherz, HZ; Giaconia, RM (1996). "The long-term sequelae of child and adolescent abuse: a longitudinal community study". *Child abuse & neglect* **20** (8): 709–23. doi:10.1016/0145-2134(96)00059-2. PMID 8866117.

[43] Bourgeois, JP (2005). "Brain synaptogenesis and epigenesis". *Médecine/Sciences* **21** (4): 428–33. doi:10.1051/medsci/2005214428. PMID 15811309.

[44] Childhood Experience and the Expression of Genetic Potential: What childhood neglect tells about nature versus nurture. Perry, BD. (2002) Article (http://www.childtrauma.org/CTAMATERIALS/MindBrain.pdf)

[45] Weaver, IC; Cervoni, N; Champagne, FA; D'alessio, AC; Sharma, S; Seckl, JR; Dymov, S; Szyf, M et al (2004). "Epigenetic programming by maternal behavior". *Nature neuroscience* **7** (8): 847–54. doi:10.1038/nn1276. PMID 15220929.

[46] McGowan, PO; Sasaki, A; D'alessio, AC; Dymov, S; Labonté, B; Szyf, M; Turecki, G; Meaney, MJ (2009). "Epigenetic regulation of the glucocorticoid receptor in human brain associates with childhood abuse". *Nature neuroscience* **12** (3): 342–8. doi:10.1038/nn.2270. PMC 2944040. PMID 19234457.

[47] Meaney, MJ; Szyf, M (2005). "Environmental programming of stress responses through DNA methylation: life at the interface between a dynamic environment and a fixed genome". *Dialogues in clinical neuroscience* **7** (2): 103–23. PMC 3181727. PMID 16262207.

[48] Skinner, MK; Anway, MD; Savenkova, MI; Gore, AC; Crews, D; Baune, Bernhard (2008). Baune, Bernhard. ed. "Transgenerational epigenetic programming of the brain transcriptome and anxiety behavior". *PloS one* **3** (11): e3745. doi:10.1371/journal.pone.0003745. PMC 2581440. PMID 19015723.

[49] Whitelaw, NC; Whitelaw, E (2006). "How lifetimes shape epigenotype within and across generations". *Human molecular genetics* **15 Spec No 2**: R131–7. doi:10.1093/hmg/ddl200. PMID 16987876.

[50] Skinner, MK; Manikkam, M; Guerrero-Bosagna, C (2010). "Epigenetic transgenerational actions of environmental factors in disease etiology". *Trends in endocrinology and metabolism: TEM* **21** (4): 214–22. doi:10.1016/j.tem.2009.12.007. PMC 2848884. PMID 20074974.

[51] Bohnen, N; Nicolson, N; Sulon, J; Jolles, J (1991). "Coping style, trait anxiety and cortisol reactivity during mental stress". *Journal of psychosomatic research* **35** (2–3): 141–7. doi:10.1016/0022-3999(91)90068-Y. PMID 2046048.

[52] Yehuda, R; Bierer, LM (2008). "Transgenerational transmission of cortisol and PTSD risk". *Progress in brain research* **167**: 121–35. doi:10.1016/S0079-6123(07)67009-5. PMID 18037011.

[53] Neigh, GN; Gillespie, CF; Nemeroff, CB (2009). "The neurobiological toll of child abuse and neglect". *Trauma, violence & abuse* **10** (4): 389–410. doi:10.1177/1524838009339758. PMID 19661133.

[54] Weaver, IC; Champagne, FA; Brown, SE; Dymov, S; Sharma, S; Meaney, MJ; Szyf, M (2005). "Reversal of maternal programming of stress responses in adult offspring through methyl supplementation: altering epigenetic marking later in life". *Journal of Neuroscience* **25** (47): 11045–54. doi:10.1523/JNEUROSCI.3652-05.2005. PMID 16306417.

[55] Kalin, JH; Butler, KV; Kozikowski, AP (2009). "Creating zinc monkey wrenches in the treatment of epigenetic disorders". *Current opinion in chemical biology* **13** (3): 263–71. doi:10.1016/j.cbpa.2009.05.007. PMID 19541531.

[56] Weaver, IC; Meaney, MJ; Szyf, M (2006). "Maternal care effects on the hippocampal transcriptome and anxiety-mediated behaviors in the offspring that are reversible in adulthood". *Proceedings of the National Academy of Sciences of the United States of America* **103** (9): 3480–5. doi:10.1073/pnas.0507526103. PMC 1413873. PMID 16484373.

[57] "NIMH · Post Traumatic Stress Disorder Research Fact Sheet" (http://www.nimh.nih.gov/health/publications/post-traumatic-stress-disorder-research-fact-sheet/index.shtml). *National Institutes of Health*. .

[58] Dubner, AE; Motta, RW (1999). "Sexually and physically abused foster care children and posttraumatic stress disorder". *Journal of consulting and clinical psychology* **67** (3): 367–73. doi:10.1037/0022-006X.67.3.367. PMID 10369057.

[59] Casey Family Programs, Harvard Medical School (2005.04.05). "Former Foster Children in Oregon and Washington Suffer Posttraumatic Stress Disorder at Twice the Rate of U.S War Veterans" Jimcaseyyouth.org (http://www.jimcaseyyouth.org/docs/nwa_release.pdf). Retrieved 2010.03.23.

[60] Cook, Rebecca (2005-04-07). "One in four foster children suffers from post-traumatic stress, study finds" (http://seattletimes.nwsource.com/html/health/2002232816_webptsd06.html). Seattletimes.nwsource.com. . Retrieved 2011-11-01.

[61] Hadfield, SC; Preece, PM (2008). "Obesity in looked after children: is foster care protective from the dangers of obesity?". *Child: care, health and development* **34** (6): 710–2. doi:10.1111/j.1365-2214.2008.00874.x. PMID 18959567.

[62] Gilmour, J; Skuse, D; Pembrey, M (2001). "Hyperphagic short stature and Prader—Willi syndrome: a comparison of behavioural phenotypes, genotypes and indices of stress". *The British journal of psychiatry : the journal of mental science* **179** (2): 129–37. doi:10.1192/bjp.179.2.129. PMID 11483474.

[63] Skuse, D; Albanese, A; Stanhope, R; Gilmour, J; Voss, L (1996). "A new stress-related syndrome of growth failure and hyperphagia in children, associated with reversibility of growth-hormone insufficiency". *Lancet* **348** (9024): 353–8. doi:10.1016/S0140-6736(96)01358-X. PMID 8709732.

[64] Demb, JM (1991). "Reported hyperphagia in foster children". *Child abuse & neglect* **15** (1–2): 77–88. doi:10.1016/0145-2134(91)90092-R. PMID 2029675.

[65] "Northwest Foster Care Alumni Study" (http://research.casey.org). Research.casey.org. . Retrieved 2011-11-01.

[66] Carlson, V., Cicchetti, D., Barnett, D., & Braunwald, K. (1995). Finding order in disorganization: Lessons from research on maltreated infants' attachments to their caregivers. In D. Cicchetti & V. Carlson (Eds), Child Maltreatment: Theory and research on the causes and consequences of child abuse and neglect (pp. 135–157). NY: Cambridge University Press.

[67] Cicchetti, D., Cummings, E.M., Greenberg, M.T., & Marvin, R.S. (1990). An organizational perspective on attachment beyond infancy. In M. Greenberg, D. Cicchetti, & M. Cummings (Eds), Attachment in the Preschool Years (pp. 3–50). Chicago: University of Chicago Press.

[68] Gauthier, L., Stollak, G., Messe, L., & Arnoff, J. (1996). Recall of childhood neglect and physical abuse as differential predictors of current psychological functioning. Child Abuse and Neglect 20, 549–559

[69] Malinosky-Rummell, R.; Hansen, D.J. (1993). "Long term consequences of childhood physical abuse". *Psychological Bulletin* **114** (1): 68–69. doi:10.1037/0033-2909.114.1.68. PMID 8346329.

[70] Lyons-Ruth K. & Jacobvitz, D. (1999) Attachment disorganization: unresolved loss, relational violence and lapses in behavioral and attentional strategies. In J. Cassidy & P. Shaver (Eds.) Handbook of Attachment. (pp. 520–554). Publisher: The Guilford Press; 1 edition (August 13, 1999) Language: English ISBN 1-57230-480-4 ISBN 978-1-57230-480-2

[71] Greenberg, M. (1999). Attachment and Psychopathology in Childhood. In J. Cassidy & P. Shaver (Eds.). Handbook of Attachment (pp.469–496). NY: Guilford Press

[72] Solomon, J. & George, C. (Eds.) (1999). Attachment Disorganization. Publisher: The Guilford Press; 1 edition (August 13, 1999) Language: English ISBN 1-57230-480-4 ISBN 978-1-57230-480-2

[73] Main, M. & Hesse, E. (1990) Parents' Unresolved Traumatic Experiences are related to infant disorganized attachment status. In M.T. Greenberg, D. Ciccehetti, & E. M. Cummings (Eds), Attachment in the Preschool Years: Theory, Research, and Intervention (pp161-184). Chicago: University of Chicago Press

[74] Carlson, E. A. (1988). "A prospective longitudinal study of disorganized/disoriented attachment". *Child Development* **69** (4): 1107–1128. PMID 9768489.

[75] Lyons-Ruth, K. (1996). "Attachment relationships among children with aggressive behavior problems: The role of disorganized early attachment patterns". *Journal of Consulting and Clinical Psychology* **64** (1): 64–73. doi:10.1037/0022-006X.64.1.64. PMID 8907085.

[76] Lyons-Ruth, K.; Alpern, L.; Repacholi, B. (1993). "Disorganized infant attachment classification and maternal psychosocial problems as predictors of hostile-aggressive behavior in the preschool classroom". *Child Development* **64** (2): 572–585. doi:10.2307/1131270. JSTOR 1131270. PMID 8477635.

[77] "Throwaway kids" (http://www.pasadenaweekly.com/article.php?id=3559&IssueNum=25). Pasadena Weekly. 2006-06-22. . Retrieved 2011-11-01.

[78] "Saving foster kids from the streets / As the nation faces a new wave of homeless children, Larkin youth center helps provide a transition to adulthood" (http://sfgate.com/cgi-bin/article.cgi?f=/c/a/2004/04/11/MNGPH63KM31.DTL). Sfgate.com. 2004-04-11. . Retrieved 2011-11-01.

[79] Current Controversies: Issues in Adoption. Ed. William Dudley. Publisher: Greenhaven Press; 1 edition (December 19, 2003) Language: English ISBN 0-7377-1626-6 ISBN 978-0-7377-1626-9

[80] Lopez, P; Allen, PJ (2007). "Addressing the health needs of adolescents transitioning out of foster care". *Pediatric nursing* **33** (4): 345–55. PMID 17907736.

[81] V.Roman, N.P. & Wolfe, N. (1995). Web of failure: The relationship between foster care and homelessness. Washington, DC: National Alliance to End Homelessness.

[82] "80 Percent Failure A Brief Analysis of the Casey Family Programs Northwest Foster Care Alumni Study" (http://nccpr.info/80-percent-failure/). Nccpr.info. 2005-04-07. . Retrieved 2011-11-01.

[83] Web of Failure: The Relationship Between Foster Care and Homelessness, Nan P. Roman, Phyllis Wolfe, National Alliance to End Homelessness

[84] Charles, G; Matheson, J (1991). "Suicide prevention and intervention with young people in foster care in Canada". *Child welfare* **70** (2): 185–91. PMID 2036873.

[85] "Improving Outcomes for Older Youth" (http://www.casey.org/Resources/Publications/pdf/WhitePaper_ImprovingOutcomesOlderYouth_FR.pdf) (PDF). . Retrieved 2011-11-01.

[86] Vinnerljung, B; Hjern, A; Lindblad, F (2006). "Suicide attempts and severe psychiatric morbidity among former child welfare clients—a national cohort study". *Journal of child psychology and psychiatry, and allied disciplines* **47** (7): 723–33. doi:10.1111/j.1469-7610.2005.01530.x. PMID 16790007.

[87] Barth, R (1998). "Death rates among California's foster care and former foster care populations". *Children and Youth Services Review* **20** (7): 577–604. doi:10.1016/S0190-7409(98)00027-9.

[88] Kalland, M; Pensola, TH; MerilÃ¤inen, J; Sinkkonen, J (2001). "Mortality in children registered in the Finnish child welfare registry: population based study". *BMJ (Clinical research ed.)* **323** (7306): 207–8. doi:10.1136/bmj.323.7306.207. PMC 35273. PMID 11473912.

[89] "The Corrupt Business of Child Protective Services – report by Senator Nancy Schaefer, September 25, 2008" (http://www.nccr.info/attachments/600_The Corrupt Business Of Child Protective Services.pdf). .

[90] "Findings from the Northwest Foster Care Alumni Study" (http://www.casey.org/Resources/Publications/pdf/ImprovingFamilyFosterCare_FR.pdf). .

[91] *Unfulfilled Promise: The Dimensions and Characteristics of Philadelphia's Dropout Crisis, 2000–05," JHU.edu (http://www.csos.jhu.edu/new/Neild_Balfanz_06.pdf)

[92] "Incarnation Controversy Simmers: City's Agency Handling of HIV Kids Still Questioned by Foster Parents" (http://www.indypendent.org/?p=532). The Indypendent. 2005-12-08. . Retrieved 2011-11-01.

[93] Zito, JM; Safer, DJ; Sai, D; Gardner, JF; Thomas, D; Coombes, P; Dubowski, M; Mendez-Lewis, M (2008). "Psychotropic medication patterns among youth in foster care". *Pediatrics* **121** (1): e157–63. doi:10.1542/peds.2007-0212. PMID 18166534.

[94] Psychiatry (Edgmont). 2008 April; 5(4): 25–26. Full text at PMC: 2719553 (http://www.ncbi.nlm.nih.gov/pmc/articles/PMC2719553/) Elisa F. Cascade and Amir H. Kalali, MD

[95] Hobbs, GF; Hobbs, CJ; Wynne, JM (1999). "Abuse of children in foster and residential care". *Child abuse & neglect* **23** (12): 1239–52. doi:10.1016/S0145-2134(99)00096-4. PMID 10626608.

[96] "Law Article – Law Related Articles" (http://www.hg.org/article.asp?id=6703). Hg.org. . Retrieved 2011-11-01.

[97] "Foster Care vs. Family Preservation" (http://www.nccpr.org/reports/01SAFETY.pdf). .

[98] Pecora, Peter J.. "Improving Family Foster Care | Casey Family Programs" (http://www.casey.org/Resources/Publications/ImprovingFamilyFosterCare.htm). Casey.org. . Retrieved 2011-11-01.

[99] "South Bay sex-abuse lawsuit: Ex-foster child awarded $30 million – San Jose Mercury News" (http://www.mercurynews.com/ci_15684415?nclick_check=1). Mercurynews.com. . Retrieved 2011-11-01.

[100] "Estey & Bomberger announces Jury Awards $30 Million in San Jose Molestation Case" (http://www.businesswire.com/news/home/20100805006437/en/Estey-Bomberger-announces-Jury-Awards-30-Million). .

[101] Aimee Green, The Oregonian. "Gresham foster kids abused despite DHS checks" (http://www.oregonlive.com/news/index.ssf/2009/04/gresham_foster_kids_abused_des.html). OregonLive.com. . Retrieved 2011-11-01.

[102] Michelle Cole, The Oregonian. "Abuse in children's foster care: State officials call for outside review" (http://www.oregonlive.com/politics/index.ssf/2009/09/abuse_in_foster_care_state_off.html). OregonLive.com. . Retrieved 2011-11-01.

[103] "Foster Care Child Molestation, Department of Children & Families pays $175,000 negligence settlement" (http://www.lawyersandsettlements.com/settlements/10747/foster-care-child-molestation.html). Lawyersandsettlements.com. . Retrieved 2011-11-01.

[104] "Foster parent, 79, accused of molesting girls in his care" (http://cftlaw.com/news.php?category=Firm+In+the+News&headline=Lawsuits+against+Department+of+Children+&+Families+cost+state+$2.26+million). .

[105] Swift, Aisling. "Child of rape now 9, yet DCF settlement held up » Naples Daily News" (http://www.naplesnews.com/news/2009/mar/27/child-rape-now-9-yet-dcf-settlement-held/). Naplesnews.com. . Retrieved 2011-11-01.

[106] "Florida Committee Substitute for Senate Bill No. 60" (http://laws.flrules.org/2010/235). .

[107] http://www.flsenate.gov/data/session/2010/Senate/bills/billtext/pdf/s0060.pdf

[108] "Charlie and Nadine H. v. McGreevey" (http://www.youthlaw.org/publications/fc_docket/alpha/charlieandnadineh/). Youthlaw.org. . Retrieved 2011-11-01.

[109] "New Jersey (Charlie and Nadine H. v. Christie) — Children's Rights" (http://www.childrensrights.org/reform-campaigns/legal-cases/new-jersey-charlie-and-nadine-h-v-corzine/). Childrensrights.org. . Retrieved 2011-11-01.

[110] "Charlie and Nadine H. v. Codey, also known as Charlie and Nadine H. v. McGreevey and Charlie and Nadine H. v. Whitman : National Center for Youth Law" (http://www.youthlaw.org/publications/fc_docket/alpha/charlieandnadineh/). youthlaw.org. . Retrieved 2011-11-01.

[111] "Legal Documents(Charlie and Nadine H. v. Corzine)" (http://www.childrensrights.org/reform-campaigns/legal-cases/new-jersey-charlie-and-nadine-h-v-corzine/2/). .

[112] Home Reform Campaigns Results of Reform Results of Reform. "Results of Reform — Children's Rights" (http://www.childrensrights.org/reform-campaigns/results-of-reform/). Childrensrights.org. . Retrieved 2011-11-01.

[113] The Daily Mail: " Paedophile with a long history of abuse was able to foster a child after council failures (http://www.dailymail.co.uk/news/article-1384180/Convicted-paedophile-allowed-foster-child-major-council-blunder-meant-checks-werent-carried-out.html)", May 6, 2011. Retrieved December 28, 2011.

[114] BBC: " Foster carer Patrick Gallagher jailed for child sex abuse (http://www.bbc.co.uk/news/uk-england-nottinghamshire-13527480)", May 24, 2011. Retrieved December 28, 2011.

[115] http://fostercareinjustice.wordpress.com/2011/11/06/who-gives-the-more-sensual-search-the-tsa-or-macomb-county-youth-home/

[116] Johansen-Berg, H (2007). "Structural plasticity: rewiring the brain". *Current biology : CB* **17** (4): R141–4. doi:10.1016/j.cub.2006.12.022. PMID 17307051.

[117] Duffau, H (2006). "Brain plasticity: from pathophysiological mechanisms to therapeutic applications". *Journal of Clinical Neuroscience* **13** (9): 885–97. doi:10.1016/j.jocn.2005.11.045. PMID 17049865.

[118] Holtmaat, A; Svoboda, K (2009). "Experience-dependent structural synaptic plasticity in the mammalian brain". *Nature reviews. Neuroscience* **10** (9): 647–58. doi:10.1038/nrn2699. PMID 19693029.

[119] Ge, S; Sailor, KA; Ming, GL; Song, H (2008). "Synaptic integration and plasticity of new neurons in the adult hippocampus". *The Journal of physiology* **586** (16): 3759–65. doi:10.1113/jphysiol.2008.155655. PMC 2538931. PMID 18499723.

[120] Chen CY, Gerhard T, Winterstein AG. Determinants of initial pharmacological treatment for youths with attention-deficit/hyperactivity disorder. J Child Adolesc Psychopharmacol. 2009 Apr;19(2):187-95. PMID 19364296

[121] Weinstein, D; Staffelbach, D; Biaggio, M (2000). "Attention-deficit hyperactivity disorder and posttraumatic stress disorder: differential diagnosis in childhood sexual abuse". *Clinical psychology review* **20** (3): 359–78. doi:10.1016/S0272-7358(98)00107-X. PMID 10779899.

[122] Becker-Weidman, A., & Shell, D., (Eds.) Creating Capacity for Attachment, Oklahoma City, OK: Wood N Barnes, 2005/2009/2011

[123] Becker-Weidman, A., Dyadic Developmental Psychotherapy: Essential Methods & Practices, Jason Aronson, Lanham, MD, 2010

[124] Hughes, D., Attachment Focused Family Therapy, Norton: NY, 2009

[125] *Adoption Detective: Memoir of an Adopted Child*, Judith and Martin Land, (2011), Chapter 5—Foster Parents, p. 20-26, Epilogue, p. 259-260, and References p. 275

[126] Bones Season 4 *TOP 10 Most Shocking Moments* (http://boneswiki.fox.com/page/Best+of+Bones+Season+4)

[127] Secret Life Of The American Teenager *Margaret* (http://abcfamily.go.com/abcfamily/path/section_Shows+Secret-Life-Of-The-American-Teenager/page_LScott-Caldwell)

[128] "The Leverage Team – Parker's Biography" (http://www.tnt.tv/series/leverage/characters/?contentId=41358). Tnt.tv. . Retrieved 2011-11-01.

[129] "The Leverage Team – Alec Hardison's Biography" (http://www.tnt.tv/series/leverage/characters/?contentId=41356). Tnt.tv. . Retrieved 2011-11-01.

[130] "Foster to Famous" (http://www.fosterclub.com/famous). Fosterclub.com. . Retrieved 2011-11-01.

Further reading

- Hurley, Kendra (2002). "Almost Home" (http://www.nhi.org/online/issues/125/fostercare.html) Retrieved June 27, 2006.
- Carlson, E.A. (1998). "A prospective longitudinal study of disorganized/disoriented attachment". *Child Development* **69** (4): 1107–1128. PMID 9768489.
- Knowlton, Paul E. (2001). "The Original Foster Care Survival Guide"; A first person account directed to successfully aging out of foster care.
- McCutcheon, James, 2010. "Historical Analysis and Contemporary Assessment of Foster Care in Texas: Perceptions of Social Workers in a Private, Non-Profit Foster Care Agency". Applied Research Projects. Texas State University Paper 332. (http://ecommons.txstate.edu/arp/332)

External links

- The Mental Health of Children in Out-of-Home Care: Scale and Complexity of Mental Health Problems (http://www.medscape.com/viewarticle/575410_2)
- Effects of Enhanced Foster Care on the Long-term Physical and Mental Health of Foster Care Alumni (http://archpsyc.ama-assn.org/cgi/content/full/65/6/625)

Stepfamily

A **stepfamily** is a family where one parent has children that are not related to the other parent. Either one or both parents may have children from a previous relationship. Children from a stepfamily may live with one biological parent and visit their other biological parent, or they may live with each biological parent for a period of time.[1]

The traditional and strictest definition of a "stepfamily" is a married couple where one or both members of the couple have pre-existing children who live with them.[2] More recently, the definition is often expanded to include all cohabiting couples, whether married or not.[3] Some people also apply the term to non-custodial relationships, where "stepparent" can refer to the partner of a parent with whom the child does not live.[4] The term is not generally used (but can be in individual cases) to refer to the relationship with an adult child who never lived in the home with the parent's new partner.

A stepfamily can be "simple," in which only one member of the couple has a prior child or children, or it can be "complex" or "blended." In a blended stepfamily, both members of the couple may have had pre-existing children, or the couple may have additional children together. If both members of the couple have prior children, the children are stepbrothers and stepsisters to one another. Any subsequent child born to the couple becomes the half-sister or half-brother of the prior children from previous relations.

If a stepparent legally adopts the partner's child or children, he or she becomes their legal parent. In such cases they may stop using the terms "stepparent" and "stepchild" and simply refer to the child as their son or daughter. However, some of the emotional and psychological issues common to stepfamilies may still persist.

In many cases, a family member is just as bonded with his/her stepfamily as with the biological family.

Statistics

Statistics in the United States are difficult to come by, because the U.S. Census Bureau has discontinued providing estimates of marriage, divorce, and remarriage except for those that are available from the 1990 and earlier censuses.[4]

- The most common form of blended family is a mother and stepfather arrangement, since mothers often maintain custody of the children.[2]
- One-third of all children entering stepfamilies were born to an unmarried mother; the other two-thirds of cases involve divorce or the death of one parent.[5]
- Of the 60 million American children under the age of 13, half are currently living with one biological parent and that parent's current partner.[6]
- The 1990 U.S. census estimated that by the year 2000 there would be more stepfamilies than original families.[6]
- If only children residing in legally married stepfamilies are included, 23% of U.S. children would be designated as living in a stepfamily; when children are included who live with a cohabiting parent, the figure rises to 30%.[7]

Etymology

The earliest recorded use of the prefix *step-*, in the form *steop-*, is from an 8th century glossary of Latin-Old English words. *Steopsunu* is given for the Latin word *filiaster* and *steopmoder* for *nouerca*. Similar words recorded later in Old English include *stepbairn*, *stepchild* and *stepfather*. The words are used to denote a connection resulting from the remarriage of a widowed parent and are related to the word *ástíeped* meaning bereaved, with *stepbairn* and *stepchild* occasionally used simply as synonyms for *orphan*. Words such as *stepbrother*, *stepniece* and *stepparent* appeared much later and do not have any particular connotation of bereavement. Corresponding words in other Germanic languages include: Old High German *stiuf-* and Old Norse *stjúp-*.[8]

Legal status

Although, historically, stepfamilies are built through the institution of marriage, and are legally recognized, it is currently unclear if a stepfamily can be both established and recognized by less formal arrangements, such as when a man or woman with children cohabits with another man or woman outside of marriage. This relationship is becoming more common in all Western countries.

Historically and to this day, there appear to be many cultures in which these families are recognized socially as de facto families. However, in modern Western culture it is often unclear as to what, if any, social status and protection they enjoy in law.

The stepparent is a "legal stranger" in most of the U.S. and has no legal right to the minor child no matter how involved in the child's life they are. The biological parents (and, where applicable, adoptive parents) hold that privilege and responsibility. So if the biological parent doesn't give up his or her parental rights and custody of the child, the other parent's subsequent marriage cannot create a parental relationship without the biological parent's written consent before a "child" reaches adulthood. In most cases, the stepparent can not be ordered to pay child support.

With regard to unmarried couples, one can easily imagine such social and legal recognition, most notably in the case of common law marriage. Unmarried couples today may also find social recognition locally through community consensus.

Still, it is not at all clear what formal parenting roles, rights, responsibilities and social etiquette should exist between "stepparents" and their "stepchildren." This often leaves the parents in unexpected conflicts with each other, their former spouses and the children.

For all the confusion which stepparents may feel, it is often even less clear to the stepchildren what the interpersonal relationships are, or should be, between themselves and their stepsiblings; between themselves and their stepparent; and even between themselves and their birth parents. These relationships can be extremely complex, especially in circumstances where each "stepspouse" may bring children of their own to the home or in households where children are expected to actively participate in each of the newly created families of both birth parents.

Although most stepfamilies can agree on what they do not want to be for one another, they are often hard pressed to agree upon what they do want to be for one another. This makes it difficult for everyone in the family to learn their roles. It is especially difficult for the children, because the roles and expectations of them change as they move between the homes and families of both of their birth parents.

Stepparent adoption

Stepparents can become legal parents to their stepchildren through the process of stepparent adoption. *Both* biological parents, if living, must consent or agree to the adoption. When a stepparent adopts a stepchild, either the non-custodial parent of the child willingly gives up his or her parental rights to the child, or the court terminates the parental rights of a biological parent if there is evidence of abuse or neglect to the child. If a parent is not involved in the child's life, the court can terminate that biological parent's rights on the grounds of abandonment. Grounds for abandonment in most states are no contact between the parent and child for at least one year.

It is important to check with local laws when looking to complete a stepparent adoption. While having the non-custodial parent consent to the adoption is the easiest way to complete a stepparent adoption, it is still possible to have one completed when they either do not consent, or cannot be located.

If the biological parent who is not involved in the child's life cannot be found, a stepparent adoption can still occur. Typically, a public notice must be published in the newspaper for 30–45 days, stating the intention to have the biological parent's rights terminated, and the intent for the stepparent to adopt the child. If the biological parent does not respond to the notice, then the stepparent adoption will continue as though the absent parent consented to the adoption.

Stepparent adoption also can occur if the other biological parent is deceased.

In research

In her book, *Becoming a Stepfamily*, Patricia Papernow (1993) suggests that each stepfamily goes through seven distinct stages of development, which can be divided into the Early, Middle, and Late stages. The Early stages consist of the Fantasy, Immersion, and Awareness stages. In the Fantasy stage, both children and parents are typically "stuck" in their fantasies or wishes for what their family could be like. The developmental task for this stage is for each member to articulate their wants and needs. In the Immersion stage, the family is typically struggling to live out the fantasy of a "perfect" blended family. In this stage, it is critical for the "insider spouse" (i.e. the biological parent who typically forms the emotional hub of the family) to understand that the feelings of the "outsider spouse" and children are real. The task of this stage is to persist in the struggle to become aware of the various experiences. This stage is followed by the Awareness stage, in which the family gathers information about what the new family looks like (e.g., roles, traditions, "family culture") and how each member feels about it. The tasks of this stage are twofold: individual and joint. The individual task is for each member to begin to put words to the feelings they are experiencing, and to voice their needs to other family members. The joint task is for family members to begin to transcend the "experiential gaps" and to try to form an understanding of other members' roles and experiences.[9]

The Middle stages consist of the Mobilization and Action stages. In the Mobilization stage, the stepparent can begin to step forward to address the family's process and structure. The tasks of this stage are to confront differences in each member's perception of the new family, as well as to influence one another before shaming or blaming begins to take action to reorganize the family structure. The goal here is to make joint decisions about new stepfamily rituals, rules, and roles. The focus in this stage is on the stepfamily's unique "middle ground" (i.e. the "areas of shared experience, shared values, and easy cooperative functioning created over time," p. 39), and on balancing this new middle ground with honoring of past and other relationships.[10]

The Later stages consist of the Contact and Resolution stages. In the Contact stage, the couple is working well together, the boundaries between households are clear, and stepparents have definite roles with stepchildren as "intimate outsiders." The task for this stage is in solidifying the stepparent's role, and in continuing the process of awareness. Finally, in the Resolution stage, the stepfamily's identity has become secure. The family accepts itself for who it is, there is a strong sense of the stepfamily's middle ground, and children feel secure in both households. The task for this stage is to nourish the depth and maturity gained through this process, and to rework any issues that might arise at family "nodal events" (e.g., weddings, funerals, graduations, etc.).[11]

- Children in a one parent family often feel threatened when their parent is dating as the parent is looking for a prospective spouse. The prospective spouse can often feel threatened as the children become part of the package within the relationship. Stepfamilies can sometimes find it difficult to feel like a family as the spouse may not feel equal to the children due to the fact that a biological parent and their biological child have a stronger bond which is separate from the marriage. [12]

In fiction

Stepmothers

The notion of the word *stepmother* being descriptive of an intrinsically unkind parent is suggested by peculiar wording in John Gamble's "An Irish Wake" (1826). He writes of a woman soon to die, who instructs her successor to "be kind to my children." Gamble writes that the injunction was forgotten and that she "proved a very step-mother."

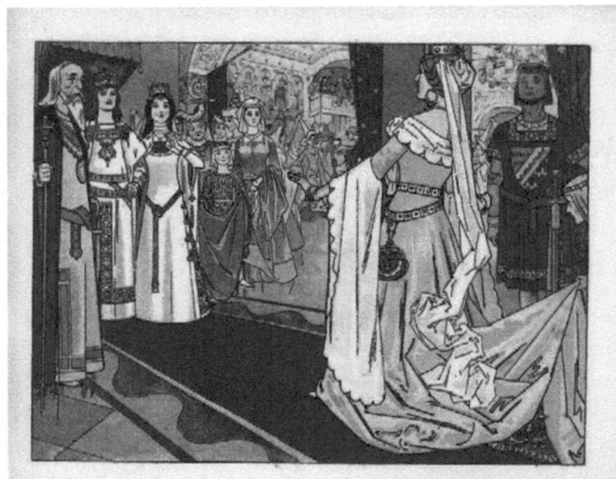

Illustration of *Schneewittchen (Snow White)* by Franz Jüttner: the evil stepmother realizes her stepdaughter has escaped her magic.

Fairy tales

In fiction, stepmothers are often portrayed as being wicked and evil.[13] The character of the wicked stepmother features heavily in fairy tales; the most famous examples are *Cinderella*, *Snow White*, and *Hansel and Gretel*. Stepdaughters are her most common victim, and then stepdaughter/stepson pairs, but stepsons also are victims as in *The Juniper Tree*[14] —sometime, as in *East of the Sun and West of the Moon*, because he refused to marry his stepsister as she wished,[15] or, indeed, they may make their stepdaughters-in-law their victims, as in *The Boys with the Golden Stars*.[16] In some fairy tales, such as Giambattista Basile's *La Gatta Cennerentola* or the Danish *Green Knight*, the stepmother wins the marriage by ingratiating herself with the stepdaughter, and once she obtains it, becomes cruel.[17]

In some fairy tales, the stepdaughter's escape by marrying does not free her from her stepmother. After the birth of the stepdaughter's first child, the stepmother may attempt to murder the new mother and replace her with her own daughter—thus making her the stepmother to the next generation. Such a replacement occurs in *The Wonderful Birch*, *Brother and Sister*, and *The Three Little Men in the Wood*; only by foiling the stepmother's plot (and usually executing her), is the story brought to a happy ending.[18] In the Korean Folktale *Janghwa Hongreyon*, the stepmother kills her own stepdaughters.

Fairy tales can have variants where one tale has an evil mother and the other an evil stepmother: in *The Six Swans*, the heroine is persecuted by her husband's mother, and in *The Twelve Wild Ducks*, by his stepmother. Sometimes this appears to be a deliberate switch: The Brothers Grimm, having put in their first editions versions of *Snow White* and *Hansel and Gretel* where the villain was the mother, altered it to a stepmother in later editions, perhaps to mitigate the story's violence.[19] The Icelandic fairy tale *The Horse Gullfaxi and the Sword Gunnfoder* features a good stepmother, who indeed aids the prince like a fairy godmother, but this figure is very rare in fairy tales.

The stepmother may be identified with other evils the characters meet. For instance, both the stepmother and the witch in *Hansel and Gretel* are deeply concerned with food, the stepmother to avoid hunger, the witch with her house built of food and her desire to eat the children, and when the children kill the witch and return home, their stepmother has mysteriously died.[20]

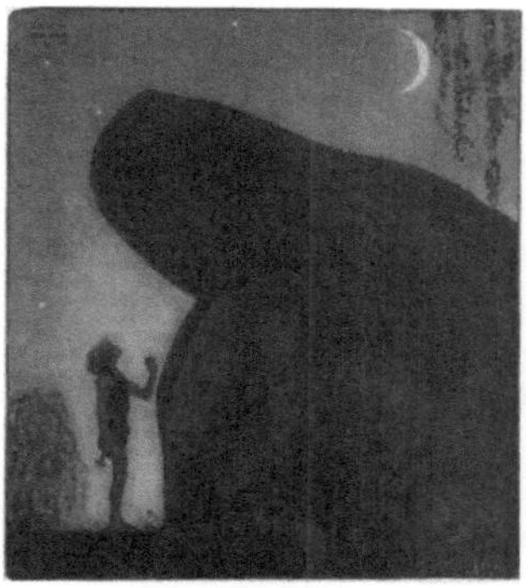

"Awake Groa Awake Mother" by John Bauer, a son at his mother's grave seeking aid against his stepmother.

In many stories with evil stepmothers, the hostility between the stepmother and the stepchild is underscored by having the child succeed through aid from the dead mother.[21] This motif occurs from Norse mythology, where Svipdagr rouses his mother Gróa from the grave so as to learn from her how to accomplish a task his stepmother set, to fairy tales such as the Brothers Grimm version of *Cinderella*, where Aschenputtel receives her clothing from a tree growing on her mother's grave, the Russian *Vasilissa the Beautiful*, where Vasilissa is aided by a doll her mother gave, and her mother's blessing, and the Malay *Bawang Putih Bawang Merah*, where the heroine's mother comes back as fish to protect her.

This hostility from the stepmother and tenderness from the true mother has been interpreted in varying ways. A psychological interpretation, by Bruno Bettelheim, describes it as "splitting" the actual mother in an ideal mother and a false mother that contains what the child dislikes in the actual mother.[22] However, historically, many women died in childbirth, their husbands remarried, and the new stepmothers competed with the children of the first marriage for resources; the tales can be interpreted as factual conflicts from history.[23] In some fairy tales, such as *The Juniper Tree*, the stepmother's hostility is overtly the desire to secure the inheritance of her children.[14]

Chinese literature

Stepmothers also make many appearances in Chinese tales of family.

Wicked stepmothers are common.[24] In *Classic of Filial Piety*, Guo Jujing told the story of Min Ziqian, who had lost his mother at a young age. His stepmother had two more sons and saw to it that they were warmly dressed in winter but neglected her stepson. When her husband discovered this, he decided to divorce her. His son interceded, on the ground that she neglected only him, but when they had no mother, all three sons would be neglected. His father relented, and the stepmother henceforth took care of all three children. For this, he was held up as a model of filial piety.

Conversely, the exemplary stepmother prefers the stepson to her own child, in recognition that his seniority makes him superior.[25] The "righteous stepmother of Qi," faced with her son and stepson having been found by a murdered man, and both having confessed to shield the other, argues for her son's execution because her husband had ordered her to look after her stepson, and her son is the junior brother; the king pardoned them both for her devotion to duty.[25]

Modern fiction

The ubiquity of the wicked stepmother has made it a frequent theme of revisionist fairy tale fantasy. This can range from Tanith Lee's *Red as Blood*, where the stepmother queen is desperately trying to protect the land from her evil stepdaughter's magic, to Diana Wynne Jones's *Howl's Moving Castle*, where, although it is known that stepmothers are evil, the actual stepmother is guilty of nothing more than some carelessness, to Erma Bombeck's retelling where Cinderella is lazy and a liar. More subtly, Piers Anthony depicted the Princess Threnody as being cursed by her stepmother in *Crewel Lye: A Caustic Yarn*: if she ever entered Castle Roogna, it would fall down. But Threnody explains that her presence at the castle caused her father to dote on her and neglect his duties to the destruction of the kingdom; her stepmother had merely made her destructive potential literal, and forced her to confront what she was doing.

Despite many examples of evil or cruel stepmothers, loving stepmothers also exist in fiction. In Kevin and Kell, Kell is portrayed as loving her stepdaughter Lindesfarne, whom her husband Kevin had adopted during his previous marriage. Likewise, Lindesfarne considers Kell her mother, and has a considerably more favorable view of her than Angelique, Kevin's ex-wife and her adoptive mother, due to feeling neglected by Angelique during her childhood. The Disney film *Enchanted* also makes references to the "evil stepmother" belief, as the villainess is a stepmother, but her wickedness comes from her selfishness and power hungriness rather than the simple fact she is a stepmother. When a little girl tells the heroine Giselle that all stepmothers are evil, Giselle reminds her that she personally knows some wonderful women who were good stepmothers, and the fact a woman is a stepmother does not suddenly change her personality. This is shown later on when Giselle gets married to that girl's father, who had her from a previous marriage, thus becoming a stepmother herself. As Giselle is a sweet and caring woman, she makes a good wife and stepmother. However, it is notable that during much of that film, Giselle was more of an older sister figure than a maternal figure to that little girl.

In the movie *Nanny McPhee* a group of children worry that their father will remarry, believing from their fairy tales that all stepmothers are an "evil breed." Although they help their father marry again to help keep the family together, their soon-to-be stepmother is very cruel, as they suspected. When the wedding to her is called off, the father decides to marry the much kinder scullery maid, causing one child to comment that the evil stepmother personification does not apply to her.

Stepmother relationships are often examined in soap operas. An example of this is the longrunning rivalry between Victoria Lord Banks and stepmother Dorian Lord on the American soap opera *One Life to Live*.

In contrast to many other Disney-related media, the cartoon show *Phineas and Ferb* features a stepfamily in which both parents get along well with their three children (avoiding the normal tropes of evil step-parents).[26]

Drake and Josh also features a stepfamily in which both parents usually get along well with their three children.

Stepfathers

Though rarer, there are also cases of evil step*fathers*, such as in the fairy tales *The Gold-bearded Man* (in a plot usually featuring a cruel father) and *The Little Bull-Calf*. One type of such tale features a defeated villain who insists on marrying the hero's mother and makes her help him trick the hero and so defeat him. Such tales include *The Prince and the Princess in the Forest* and *The Blue Belt*, although the tales of this type can also feature a different female relation, such as the stepsister in *The Three Princes and their Beasts*.

In literature, evil stepfathers include Claudius in *Hamlet* (though his role as uncle is more emphasized), Murdstone in Charles Dickens's *David Copperfield*, the classic *Twilight Zone* episode "Living Doll," the King from the movie *Radio Flyer*, and Gozaburo Kaiba (who adopted Seto and Mokuba Kaiba) from *Yu-Gi-Oh!*, as well as *The Stepfather*, films. The film, *Sucker Punch* features a sexually abusive stepfather. In a classic early episode of South Park, Stan is advised, by Bill Cosby, to "snatch up" his evil stepfather in a bear trap. http://www.southparkstudios.com/full-episodes/s02e12-clubhouses

In his opera *La Cenerentola*, Gioacchino Rossini inverted the tale of *Cinderella* to have her oppressed by her stepfather. His motive is made explicit, in that providing a dowry to Cenerentola would cut into what he can give to his own daughters.[27] An analogous male figure may also appear as a wicked uncle; like the stepmother, the father's brother may covet the child's inheritance for his own children, and so maltreat his nephews or nieces. Modern films, however, seem to cast stepfathers in a somewhat kinder light, implying honorable men who marry divorced women or single mothers make good stepfathers.

Step- and half-siblings

In fairy tales, stepsiblings and half-siblings can but need not take after their mother. In *Cinderella*, the ugly sisters are the main character's stepsisters. *Mother Hulda* also features wicked stepsisters and *The Wonderful Birch* a wicked half-sister, but *The Rose-Tree* and *The Juniper Tree* feature loving half-siblings, and *Kate Crackernuts* loving stepsisters.[28]

Many romance novels feature heroes who are the stepbrother of the heroine. The step-relationship generally stems from a marriage when the hero and heroine are at least in their adolescence.

Stepfamilies

Some family films and television sitcoms feature a stepfamily as the center premise. In many cases, the stepfamily is large and full of children causing situations such as sibling rivalry, rooming, falling in love, and getting along amongst the children as popular plotlines. The stepfamily premise dates back as far as the 1968 film *Yours, Mine and Ours*. This film gave way to a classic family television sitcom about a blended family known as *The Brady Bunch*. Some contemporary family sitcoms have made the blended family sitcom more popular with the TGIF show *Step by Step* bringing about other shows such as *Aliens in the Family*, *Life with Derek*, *Drake & Josh*, and the short lived NBC family sitcom *Something So Right*. *The Life of Riley* is a 2009 British comedy television series, shown on BBC One & BBC HD. It focuses on the lives of a blended family. *Kevin and Kell* is a comic strip that focuses on a blended family. The Disney Channel animated series *Phineas and Ferb* also prominently features a blended family, chosen by co-creator Jeff "Swampy" Marsh in part due to its underuse in children's programming, and his personal experiences growing up in such a family.[29]

Stepfamily education

The prevalence of stepfamilies has increased over the past century with the increase of divorce and remarriage. These families are unique in their experiences facing many challenges which first-married families do not. For example role ambiguity, dealing with stepchildren, and ex-spouses are only a few of the issues which are unique to these families. In response to these families' desire for assistance, stepfamily education has become an increasingly common topic among scholars and educators. Although still a relatively new facet within the marriage education realm, stepfamily education provides important information which may not be addressed in traditional marriage or relationship education curriculum. As discussed by Adler-Baeder and Higginbotham (2004)[30] a number of curricula are currently available to stepfamilies and family life educators; however, further research is needed in order to determine best-practices for the field. One way in which this gap is being filled is through the current implementation of Healthy Marriage Demonstration Grants[31] in the U.S. As part of the Deficit Reduction Act of 2005, grants for healthy marriage and responsible fatherhood, which include at-risk and diverse populations such as stepfamilies, are providing important information on the evaluation of stepfamily programs and their effectiveness in servicing stepfamilies.

See also

- Cinderella effect

Selected bibliography

- LeBey, Barbara (2004). *Remarried with Children: Ten Secrets for Successfully Blending and Extending Your Family*. New York: Bantam.
- Papernow, Patricia L. (1993). *Becoming a Stepfamily: Patterns of Development in Remarried Families*. San Francisco: Jossey-Bass.

Footnotes

[1] WebMD. "Teen Health: Living with a Stepparent" (http://teens.webmd.com/living-with-step-parent). . Retrieved 5 May 2012.

[2] "Selfhelp Magazine" (http://www.adopting.org/uni/frame.php?url=http://www.shpm.com/articles/parenting/families.html). Adopting.org. . Retrieved 2010-08-11.

[3] "adopting.org" (http://www.adopting.org/uni/frame.php?url=http://www.stepfamily.org/statistics.html). adopting.org. . Retrieved 2010-08-11.

[4] National Stepfamily Resource Center (http://www.stepfamilies.info/faqs/factsheet.php)

[5] "adopting.org, quoting the National Survey of Families and Households" (http://www.adopting.org/uni/frame.php?url=http://www.stepfamily.org/statistics.html). Adopting.org. . Retrieved 2010-08-11.

[6] "stepfamily.org, quoting the U.S. Bureau of Census" (http://www.stepfamily.org/statistics.html). Stepfamily.org. . Retrieved 2010-08-11.

[7] National Stepfamily Resource Center, quoting Bumpass, Raley, and Sweet, 1995, The changing character of stepfamilies: Implications of cohabitation and nonmarital childbearing (http://www.stepfamilies.info/faqs/factsheet.php), Demography 32, 425–436.

[8] "step-" *The Oxford English Dictionary*. 2nd ed. 1989. OED Online. Oxford University Press. 4 April 2000 < Registration required, retrieved 15 December 2006. (http://dictionary.oed.com/cgi/entry/50237101)>

[9] Papernow, Patricia L. (1993). "Becoming a Stepfamily: Patterns of Development in Remarried Families". San Francisco: Jossey-Bass.

[10] Papernow, 1993.

[11] Paernow, 1993.

[12] Fine, Mark A., U Missouri, Dept of Human Development & Family Studies, Columbia, US Kurdek, Lawrence A,, June, 1995 'Relation between marital quality and (step)parent-child relationship quality for parents and stepparents in stepfamilies', Journal of Family Psychology, Vol 9(2),. pp. 216-223, 19/05/2011, http://web.ebscohost.com.ezproxy-m.deakin.edu.au/ehost/detail?vid=3&hid=12&sid=dbc1e677-4a6a-459a-b232-5c71390a9472%40sessionmgr13&bdata=JnNpdGU9ZWhvc3QtbGl2ZQ%3d%3d#fam-9-2-216-ECDA.

[13] *The Hard Facts of the Grimms' Fairy Tales*, p. 141

[14] *The Annotated Classic Fairy Tales*, p. 161

[15] *The Annotated Classic Fairy Tales*, p. 193

[16] Warner, p. 221

[17] Warner, pp. 205–6

[18] *The Hard Facts of the Grimms' Fairy Tales*, pp. 147–8

[19] *The Hard Facts of the Grimms' Fairy Tales*, p. 36

[20] *The Annotated Classic Fairy Tales*, p. 57

[21] *The Hard Facts of the Grimms' Fairy Tales*, p. 151

[22] Warner, p. 212

[23] Warner, p. 213

[24] Mark Edward Lewis *The Early Chinese Empires: Qin and Han* p 157 ISBN 978-0-674-02477-9

[25] Mark Edward Lewis *The Early Chinese Empires: Qin and Han* p. 158 ISBN 978-0-674-02477-9

[26] http://www.bellaonline.com/articles/art8292.asp

[27] Warner, pp. 213–4

[28] *The Annotated Classic Fairy Tales*, p. 230

[29] Bond, Paul (7 June 2009). "Q&A: Dan Povenmire" (http://74.125.93.132/search?q=cache:h-TlYnF0OCMJ:www.hollywoodreporter.com/hr/content_display/news/e3i0bc78baf8235f8b4159fd786ff9f8736+Emmy+nominee+Dan+Povenmire&cd=1&hl=en&ct=clnk&gl=us&client=firefox-a). *Hollywood Reporter*. Archived from the original (http://www.hollywoodreporter.com/hr/content_display/news/e3i0bc78baf8235f8b4159fd786ff9f8736) on 2009-07-31. . Retrieved 2009-08-26.

[30] Adler-Baeder,F. & Higginbotham, B. (2004). Implications of remarriage and stepfamily formation for marriage education. *Family Relations*, 53, 448–458.

[31] "ACF Healthy Marriage Initiative: Funding Opportunities" (http://www.acf.hhs.gov/healthymarriage/funding/index.html). Acf.hhs.gov. . Retrieved 2010-08-11.

References

- Warner, Marina. *From the Beast to the Blonde: On Fairy Tales And Their Tellers*, ISBN 0-374-15901-7
- Tatar, Maria. *The Hard Facts of the Grimms' Fairy Tales*, ISBN 0-691-06722-8
- Tatar, Maria. *The Annotated Classic Fairy Tales*, ISBN 0-393-05163-3

External links

- Step Parents (http://www.dmoz.org/Home/Family/Parenting/Step_Parents/) at the Open Directory Project

Embryo_transfer

Embryo transfer	
Intervention	
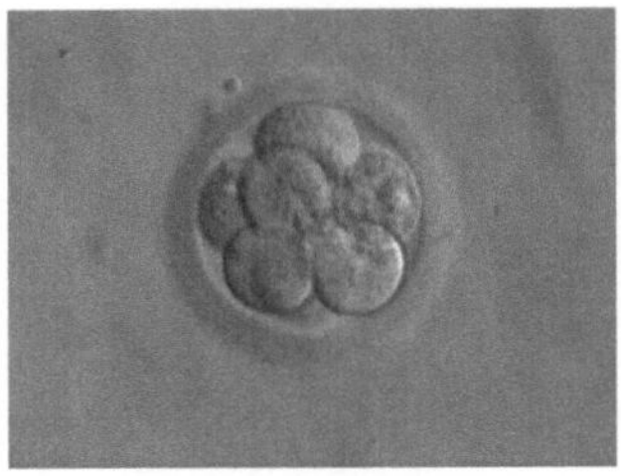 8-cell embryo for transfer 3 days after fertilization	
MeSH	D004624 [1]

Embryo transfer refers to a step in the process of assisted reproduction in which embryos are placed into the uterus of a female with the intent to establish a pregnancy. This technique (which is often used in connection with in vitro fertilization (IVF)), may be used in humans or in animals, in which situations the goals may vary.

Fresh versus frozen

Embryos can be either “fresh” from fertilized egg cells of the same menstrual cycle, or “frozen”, that is they have been generated in a preceding cycle and undergone embryo cryopreservation, and are thawed just prior to the transfer. The outcome from using cryopreserved embryos has uniformly been positive with no increase in birth defects or development abnormalities,[2] also between fresh versus frozen eggs used for intracytoplasmic sperm injection (ICSI).[3] Children born from vitrified blastocysts have significantly higher birthweight than those born from non-frozen blastocysts.[4]

Uterine preparation

In the human, the uterine lining (endometrium) needs to be appropriately prepared so that the embryo(s) can implant. In a natural or stimulated cycle, the embryo transfer takes place in the luteal phase at a time where the lining is appropriately undeveloped in relation to the status of the present Luteinizing Hormone. In a cycle where a "frozen" embryo is transferred, the recipient woman could be given first estrogen preparations (about 2 weeks), then a combination of oestrogen and progesterone so that the lining becomes receptive for the embryo. The time of receptivity is the implantation window.

Limited evidence also supports removal of cervical mucus before transfer.[5]

Timing

In stimulated cycles in human IVF, embryos are typically transferred 3 days after fertilization and may then be at the eight-cell stage, or they are transferred 2 to 3 days later when they have reached the blastocyst stage. Embryos who reach the day 3 cell stage can be tested for chromosal or specific genetic defects prior to possible transfer by preimplantation genetic diagnosis (PGD).

Monozygotic twinning is not increased after blastocyst transfer compared with cleavage-stage embryo transfer.[6]

Procedure

The embryo transfer procedure starts by placing a speculum in the vagina to visualize the cervix, which is cleansed with saline solution or culture media. A soft[5] transfer catheter is loaded with the embryos and handed to the clinician after confirmation of the patient's identity. The catheter is inserted through the cervical canal and advanced into the uterine cavity.

There is good and consistent evidence of benefit in *ultrasound guidance*,[5] that is, making an abdominal ultrasound to ensure correct placement, which is 1–2 cm from the uterine fundus. Anesthesia is generally not required. Single embryo transfers in particular require accuracy and precision in placement within the uterine cavity. The optimal target for embryo placement, known as the maximal implantation potential (MIP) point, is identified using 3D/4D ultrasound.[7] However, there is limited evidence that supports deposition of embryos in the midportion of the uterus.[5]

After insertion of the catheter, the contents are expelled and the embryos are deposited. Limited evidence supports making trial transfers before performing the procedure with embryos.[5] After expulsion, the duration that the catheter remains inside the uterus has no effect on pregnancy rates.[8] Limited evidence suggests avoiding negative pressure from the catheter after expulsion.[5] After withdrawal, the catheter is handed to the embryologist, who inspects it for retained embryos.

In the process of zygote intrafallopian transfer (ZIFT), eggs are removed from the woman, fertilised, and then placed in the woman's fallopian tubes rather than the uterus.

Embryo number

A major issue is how many embryos should be transferred. Placement of multiple embryos carries the risk of multiple pregnancy. In the past, physicians have often placed too many embryos in the hope to establish a pregnancy. However, the rise in multiple pregnancies has led to a reassessment of this approach. Professional societies and in many countries, the legislature, have issued guidelines or laws to curtail a practice of placing too many embryos in an attempt to reduce multiple pregnancies.

e-SET

The technique of selecting only one embryo to transfer to the woman is called **elective-Single Embryo Transfer (e-SET)** or, when embryos are at the blastocyst stage, it can also be called *elective single blastocyst transfer (eSBT)*.[9] It lowers the risk of multiple pregnancies, compared with e.g. Double Embryo Transfer (DET) or *double blastocyst transfer* (2BT), with a twinning rate of approximately 3.5% in sET compared with approximately 38% in DET,[10] or 2% in eSBT compared with approximately 25% in 2BT.[9] At the same time, pregnancy rates is not significantly less with eSBT than with 2BT.[9] Furthermore, SET has better outcomes in terms of mean gestational age at delivery, mode of delivery, birthweight, and risk of neonatal intensive care unit necessity than DET.[10] e-SET of embryos at the cleavage stage reduces the likelihood of live birth by 38% and multiple birth by 94%.[11] Evidence from randomized, controlled trials suggests that increasing the number of e-SET attempts (fresh and/or frozen) results in a cumulative live birth rate similar to that of DET.[11]

The usage of single embryo transfer is highest in Sweden (69.4%), but as low as 2.8% in the USA. Access to public funding for ART, availability of good cryopreservation facilities and legislation appear to be the most important factors for regional usage of single embryo transfer.[12] Also, personal choice plays a significant role as many subfertile couples have a strong preference for twins.[12]

Follow-up

Patients usually start progesterone medication after egg (also called oocyte) retrieval. While daily intramuscular injections of progesterone-in-oil (PIO) have been the standard route of administration, PIO injections are not FDA-approved for use in pregnancy. A recent meta-analysis showed that the intravaginal route with an appropriate dose and dosing frequency is equivalent to daily intramuscular injections.[13] In addition, a recent case-matched study comparing vaginal progesterone with PIO injections showed that live birth rates were nearly identical with both methods.[14] A duration of progesterone administration of 11 days results in almost the same birth rates as longer durations.[15]

Patients are also given estrogen medication in some cases after the embryo transfer. Pregnancy testing is done typically two weeks after egg retrieval.

Third-party reproduction

It is not necessary that the embryo transfer be performed on the female who provided the eggs. Thus another female whose uterus is appropriately prepared can receive the embryo and become pregnant. Embryo transfer may be used where a woman who has eggs but no uterus and wants to have a biological baby; she would require the help of a gestational carrier or surrogate to carry the pregnancy. Also, a woman who has no eggs but a uterus may resort to egg donor IVF, in which case another woman would provide eggs for fertilization and the resulting embryos are placed into the uterus of the patient. Fertilization may be performed using the woman's partner's sperm or by using donor sperm. 'Spare' embryos which are created for another couple undergoing IVF treatment but which are then surplus to that couple's needs may also be transferred (called embryo donation). Embryos may be specifically created by using eggs and sperm from donors and these can then be transferred into the uterus of another woman. A surrogate may carry a baby produced by embryo transfer for another couple, even though neither she nor the 'commissioning' couple is biologically related to the child. Third party reproduction is controversial and regulated in many countries. Persons entering gestational surrogacy arrangements must make sense of an entirely new type of relationship that does not fit any of the traditional scripts we use to categorize relations as kinship, friendship, romantic partnership or market relations.[16] Surrogates have the experience of carrying a baby that they conceptualize as not of their own kin, while intended mothers have the experience of waiting through nine months of pregnancy and transitioning to motherhood from outside of the pregnant body. This can lead to new conceptualizations of body and self.[16]

History

The first transfer of an embryo from one human to another resulting in pregnancy was reported in July 1983 and subsequently led to the announcement of the first human birth February 3, 1984.[17] This procedure was performed at the Harbor UCLA Medical Center [18] under the direction of Dr. John Buster and the University of California at Los Angeles School of Medicine.

In the procedure, an embryo that was just beginning to develop was transferred from one woman in whom it had been conceived by artificial insemination to another woman who gave birth to the infant 38 weeks later. The sperm used in the artificial insemination came from the husband of the woman who bore the baby.[19] [20]

This scientific breakthrough established standards and became an agent of change for women suffering from the afflictions of infertility and for women who did not want to pass on genetic disorders to their children. Donor embryo transfer has given women a mechanism to become pregnant and give birth to a child that will contain their husband's genetic makeup. Although donor embryo transfer as practiced today has evolved from the original non-surgical method, it now accounts for approximately 5% of in vitro fertilization recorded births.

Prior to this, thousands of women who were infertile, had adoption as the only path to parenthood. This set the stage to allow open and candid discussion of embryo donation and transfer. This breakthrough has given way to the donation of human embryos as a common practice similar to other donations such as blood and major organ donations. At the time of this announcement the event was captured by major news carriers and fueled healthy debate and discussion on this practice which impacted the future of reproductive medicine by creating a platform for further advancements in woman's health.

This work established the technical foundation and legal-ethical framework surrounding the clinical use of human oocyte and embryo donation, a mainstream clinical practice, which has evolved over the past 25 years.[19] [20] Building upon this groundbreaking research and since the initial birth announcement in 1984, well over 47,000 live births resulting from donor embryo transfer have been and continue to be recorded by the Centers for Disease Control(CDC)[21] in the United States to infertile women, who otherwise would not have had children by any other existing method.[22] [23]

Embryo transfer in animals

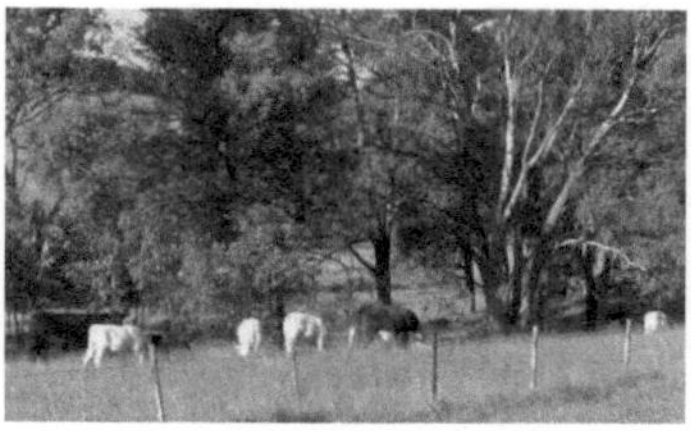

Embryo transferred Charolais calves with their Angus and Hereford recipient mothers.

Embryo transfer techniques allow top quality female livestock to have a greater influence on the genetic advancement of a herd or flock in much the same way that artificial insemination has allowed greater use of superior sires.[24] ET also allows the continued use of animals such as competition mares to continue training and showing, while producing foals. The general epidemiological aspects of embryo transfer indicates that the transfer of embryos provides the opportunity to introduce genetic material into populations of livestock while greatly reducing the risk for transmission of infectious diseases. Recent developments in the sexing of embryos before transfer and implanting has great potential in the dairy and other livestock industries.[25]

Embryo transfer is also used in laboratory mice. For example, embryos of genetically modified strains that are difficult to breed or expensive to maintain may be stored frozen, and only thawed and implanted into a pseudopregnant dam when needed.

References

[1] http://www.nlm.nih.gov/cgi/mesh/2011/MB_cgi?field=uid&term=D004624

[2] "Genetics & IVF Institute" (http://web.archive.org/web/*/http://givf.com/embryov.cfm). Givf.com. Archived from the original (http://www.givf.com/fertility/embryofreezing.cfm) on 2009-07-27. . Retrieved 2009-07-27.

[3] Error: Bad DOI specified!

[4] Wikland M, Hardarson T, Hillensjö T, *et al.* (May 2010). "Obstetric outcomes after transfer of vitrified blastocysts". *Hum Reprod* **25** (7): 1699–707. doi:10.1093/humrep/deq117. PMID 20472913.

[5] Mains L, Van Voorhis BJ (April 2010). "Optimizing the technique of embryo transfer". *Fertil Steril* **94** (3): 785–90. doi:10.1016/j.fertnstert.2010.03.030. PMID 20409543.

[6] Papanikolaou EG, Fatemi H, Venetis C, *et al.* (February 2009). "Monozygotic twinning is not increased after single blastocyst transfer compared with single cleavage-stage embryo transfer". *Fertil. Steril.* **93** (2): 592–7. doi:10.1016/j.fertnstert.2008.12.088. PMID 19243755.

[7] Gergely RZ, DeUgarte CM, Danzer H, Surrey M, Hill D, DeCherney AH (2005). "Three dimensional/four dimensional ultrasound-guided embryo transfer using the maximal implantation potential point". *Fertil. Steril.* **84** (2): 500–3. doi:10.1016/j.fertnstert.2005.01.141. PMID 16084896..

[8] Sroga JM, Montville CP, Aubuchon M, Williams DB, Thomas MA (April 2010). "Effect of delayed versus immediate embryo transfer catheter removal on pregnancy outcomes during fresh cycles". *Fertil. Steril.* **93** (6): 2088–90. doi:10.1016/j.fertnstert.2009.07.1664. PMID 20116786.

[9] Mullin CM, Fino ME, Talebian S, Krey LC, Licciardi F, Grifo JA (April 2010). "Comparison of pregnancy outcomes in elective single blastocyst transfer versus double blastocyst transfer stratified by age". *Fertil. Steril.* **93** (6): 1837–43. doi:10.1016/j.fertnstert.2008.12.137. PMID 19249756.

[10] Fauque P, Jouannet P, Davy C, *et al.* (May 2009). "Cumulative results including obstetrical and neonatal outcome of fresh and frozen-thawed cycles in elective single versus double fresh embryo transfers". *Fertil. Steril.* **94** (3): 927–35. doi:10.1016/j.fertnstert.2009.03.105. PMID 19446806.

[11] Gelbaya TA, Tsoumpou I, Nardo LG (May 2009). "The likelihood of live birth and multiple birth after single versus double embryo transfer at the cleavage stage: a systematic review and meta-analysis". *Fertil. Steril.* **94** (3): 936–45. doi:10.1016/j.fertnstert.2009.04.003. PMID 19446809.

[12] Error: Bad DOI specified!

[13] Zarutskiea PW, Phillips JA (2007). "Re-analysis of vaginal progesterone as luteal phase support (LPS) in assisted reproduction (ART) cycles". *Fertility and Sterility* **88** (supplement 1): S113. doi:10.1016/j.fertnstert.2007.07.365.

[14] Khan N, Richter KS, Blake EJ, et al. Case-matched comparison of intramuscular versus vaginal progesterone for luteal phase support after in vitro fertilization and embryo transfer. Presented at: 55th Annual Meeting of the Pacific Coast Reproductive Society; April 18–22, 2007; Rancho Mirage, CA.

[15] Goudge CS, Nagel TC, Damario MA (June 2009). "Duration of progesterone-in-oil support after in vitro fertilization and embryo transfer: a randomized, controlled trial". *Fertil. Steril.* **94** (3): 946–51. doi:10.1016/j.fertnstert.2009.05.003. PMID 19523613.

[16] Teman, Elly. 2010. Birthing a Mother: the Surrogate Body and the Pregnant Self. (http://www.ucpress.edu/books/pages/11401.php) Berkeley: University of California Press.

[17] Blakeslee, Sandra (1984-02-04). "Infertile Woman Has Baby Through Embryo Transfer" (http://query.nytimes.com/gst/fullpage.html?sec=health&res=9404EEDC143BF937A35751C0A962948260). *The New York Times*. . Retrieved 2010-05-01.

[18] http://www.humc.edu/calendar/careacc.html

[19] Friedrich, Otto; Constable, Anne; Samghabadi, Raji (1984-09-10). "Medicine: A Legal, Moral, Social Nightmare" (http://www.time.com/time/magazine/article/0,9171,952517,00.html). *Time*. . Retrieved 2010-05-01.

[20] "The New Origins of Life" (http://www.time.com/time/magazine/article/0,9171,952514,00.html). *Time*. 1984-09-10. . Retrieved 2010-05-01.

[21] http://www.cdc.gov/ART/

[22] http://www.obgmanagement.com/srm/pdf/first_live_birth_donation.pdf

[23] http://www.obgmanagement.com/srm.asp?id=5030

[24] Embryo Transfer in Cattle (http://jobfunctions.bnet.com/abstract.aspx?docid=118654) Retrieved on 21 October 2008

[25] Embryo Sexing Technology (http://www.agnet.org/library/tb/151b/) Retrieved on 21 October 2008

External links

- How embryo transfer works as part of fertility treatment (http://www.hfea.gov.uk/543.html)
- The blastocyst transfer process - a form of embryo transfer (http://www.hfea.gov.uk/544.html)
- One at a time website - benefits of Single Embryo Transfer (http://www.oneatatime.org.uk)

Egg_donation

Egg donation	
Intervention	
MeSH	D018587 [1]

Egg donation is the process by which a woman provides one or several (usually 10-15) eggs (ova, oocytes) for purposes of assisted reproduction or biomedical research. For assisted reproduction purposes, egg donation involves the process of in vitro fertilization as the eggs are fertilized in the laboratory. Egg donation is part of the process of third party reproduction as part of ART (Assisted Reproductive Technology). The ASRM (American Society of Reproductive Medicine) has issued guidelines for these procedures, and the FDA has a number of guidelines as well. There are boards in countries outside of the US who have the same regulations.

History

The first transfer of a fertilized egg from one human to another resulting in pregnancy was reported in July 1983 and subsequently led to the announcement of the first egg-donation-produced human birth on February 3, 1984.[2] This procedure was performed at the Harbor UCLA Medical Center under the direction of Dr. John Buster and the University of California at Los Angeles School of Medicine.[3]

In the procedure, a fertilized egg that was just beginning to develop was transferred from one woman in whom it had been conceived by artificial insemination to another woman who gave birth to the infant 38 weeks later. The sperm used in the artificial insemination came from the husband of the woman who bore the baby.[4] [5]

This scientific breakthrough established standards and changed the outlook for those who were unable to have children due to infertility or were at high risk for passing on genetic disorders. Donor oocytes and embryo transfer has given women a mechanism to become pregnant and give birth to a child that will be their biological child, but not their genetic child (assuming that the recipient woman carries the baby.) In many cases, a gestational surrogate is used, and the embryos are implanted into her, per an agreement with the recipients. Oocyte and embryo donation as practiced today now accounts for approximately 5% of in vitro fertilization recorded births.

Another beneficiary of this technology is the gay parent community. Surrogacy has enabled homosexual people to have biological children.

Prior to this, thousands of women who were infertile, single men and gay couples had adoption as the only path to parenthood. This set the stage to allow open and candid discussion of oocyte and embryo donation as a common practice.[4] [5] This breakthrough has given way to the donation of human oocytes and embryos as a common practice similar to other donations such as blood and major organ donations. At the time of this announcement the event was captured by major news carriers and fueled healthy debate and discussion on this practice which impacted the future of reproductive medicine by creating a platform for further advancements in woman's health.

This work established the technical foundation and legal-ethical framework surrounding the clinical use of human oocyte and embryo donation, a mainstream clinical practice, which has evolved over the past 25 years.[4] [6] Building upon this groundbreaking research and since the initial birth announcement in 1984, well over 47,000 live births resulting from donor oocyte embryo transfer have been and continue to be recorded by the Centers for Disease Control (CDC)[7] [8] in the United States to infertile women, who otherwise would not have had children by any other existing method.

The process is done today in other countries as well, but many couples come to the U.S. due to laws in many other countries which severely limit or prohibit compensation given to an egg donor. Since this process is so invasive (much more so than its counterpart, sperm donation), the lack of compensation results in an extreme dearth of young women willing to go through this procedure.

Indication

A need for egg donation may arise for a number of reasons. Infertile couples may resort to acquiring eggs through egg donation when the female partner cannot have genetic children because she may not have eggs that can generate a viable pregnancy. This situation is often, but not always based on advanced reproductive age. Early onset of menopause which can occur in women as early as their 30's can require a woman to use donor eggs to grow her family. Some women are born without ovaries or other reproductive organs. Sometimes a woman's reproductive organs have been damaged due to disease or circumstances required her to have them surgically removed. Another indication would be a genetic disorder on part of the woman that can be circumvented by using eggs from another person. Many women have none of these issues, but continue to be unsuccessful using their own eggs.

If desired, (and if the egg donor agrees), the couple can personally get acquainted with the egg donor, her children and family members. More often, egg donations are anonymous. As stated above, egg donation is also helpful for gay male couples using surrogacy (see LGBT parenting).

- **Congenital absence of eggs**
  - Turner syndrome
  - Gonadal dysgenesis
- **Acquired reduced egg quantity / quality**
  - Oophorectomy
  - Premature menopause
  - Chemotherapy
  - Radiation therapy
  - Autoimmunity
  - Advanced maternal age
  - Compromised ovarian reserve
- **Other**
  - Diseases of X-Sex linkage
  - Repetitive fertilization or pregnancy failure
  - Ovaries inaccessible for egg retrieval

Types of donors

Donors includes the following types:

- Donors unrelated to the recipients who do it for altruistic or monetary reasons. They are often *anonymous donors* typically recruited by *egg donor agencies* or, sometimes, IVF programs.
- **Designated donors**, e.g. a friend or relative brought by the patients to serve as a donor specifically to help them. In Sweden, couples who can bring such a donor still get another person as a donor, but instead get advanced on the waiting list for the procedure, and that donor rather becomes a "cross donor".[9]
- Patients taking part in **shared oocyte programmes**. Women who go through in vitro fertilization may be willing to donate unused eggs to such a program, where the egg recipients together help paying the cost of the In Vitro Fertilisation (IVF) procedure.[10] It is very cost-effective compared to other alternatives.[11] The pregnancy rates with use of shared oocytes is similar to that with altruistic donors.[12]

Procedure

Egg donors are first recruited, screened, and give consent prior to participation in the IVF process. Once the egg donor is recruited, she undergoes IVF stimulation therapy, followed by the egg retrieval procedure. After retrieval, the ova are fertilized by the sperm of the male partner (or sperm donor) in the laboratory, and, after several days, the best resulting embryo(s) is/are placed in the uterus of the recipient, whose uterine lining has been appropriately prepared for embryo transfer beforehand. The recipient is usually, but not always, the person who requested the service and then will carry and deliver the pregnancy and keep the baby.

The egg donor's process in detail

Each egg donor is required to undergo a thorough medical examination, including a pelvic exam, blood draw to check hormone levels and to test for infectious diseases, and an ultrasound to examine her ovaries, uterus and other pelvic organs. In addition, she will be referred to a psychologist who will evaluate if she is mentally prepared to undertake and complete the donation process. These evaluations are necessary to ensure that the donor is fully prepared and capable of completing the donation cycle safely and successfully.[13]

Once the screening is complete and a legal contract signed, the donor will begin the donation cycle, which typically takes between three and six weeks. An egg retrieval procedure comprises both the **Egg Donor's Cycle** and the **Recipient's Cycle**. Birth control pills are administered during the first few weeks of the egg donation[14] process to synchronize the donor's cycle with the recipient's, followed by a series of injections which halt the normal functioning of the donor's ovaries. These injections may be self-administered on a daily basis for a period of one to three weeks. Next, follicle-stimulating hormones (FSH) are given to the donor to stimulate egg production and increases the number of mature eggs produced by the ovaries. Throughout the cycle the donor is monitored often by a physician using blood tests and ultrasound exams to determine the donor's reaction to the hormones and the progress of follicle growth.[13]

Once the doctor decides the follicles are mature, he/she will establish the date and time for the egg retrieval procedure. Approximately 36 hours before retrieval, the donor must administer one last injection of HCG hormone to ensure that her eggs are ready to be harvested. The egg retrieval itself is a minimally invasive surgical procedure lasting 20–30 minutes, performed under sedation. A small ultrasound-guided needle is inserted through the vagina to aspirate the follicles in both ovaries, which extracts the eggs. After resting in a recovery room for an hour or two, the donor is released. Most donors resume regular activities by the next day.[13]

Results

Nationwide, egg donor cycles have a success rate of upwards of 60%. (See SART statistics at http://www.sart.org.) When a "fresh cycle" is followed by a "frozen cycle", the success rate with donor eggs goes up to approximately 80%. With egg donation, women who are past their reproductive years or menopause can become pregnant.

The oldest woman thus to give birth is Adriana Iliescu, age 66.

Babies born after egg donation are not genetically related to the recipient.

Donor motivation

An egg donor may be motivated by a number of reasons to provide eggs. Some egg donors may be altruistic and feel that participation in the reproductive process provides a benefit for another person, sometimes a person they know or are related to. A survey of 80 American women showed that 30% were motivated by altruism alone. Others, 20%, were attracted only by monetary compensation, while 40% of donors were motivated by both reasons. The same study reported that 45% of egg donors were students the first time they donated and averaged $4,000 for each donation.[15] In the European Union the standard for reimbursement is based on compensation, not payment limiting egg donation to, at most, $1500. In some countries, most notably Spain and Cyprus this has limited donors to the poorest segments of society.[16] Egg-recruitment agencies are known for advertising to college students in publications such-as campus newspapers. Although it is against the terms of service, egg-harvesters consistently post and re-post ads on Craigslist. That practice speaks to the integrity of the advertiser, and potential donors are warned to avoid transactions with businesses that place ads in that manner.

Risks

Egg donor

Egg donation carries risks for both donor and recipient, although it must be made clear that the procedure for the donor, and the medication given, is basically the same as the medication given for any IVF procedure (with or without a donor). The egg donor may suffer complications from IVF, such as bleeding from the oocyte recovery procedure and reaction to the hormones used to induce hyperovulation (producing more than one egg), including ovarian hyperstimulation syndrome (OHSS) and, rarely, liver failure.[17]

According to Jansen and Tucker, writing in the same ART (assisted reproductive technologies) textbook referenced above,[17] the risk of OHSS varies with the clinic administering the hormones, from 6.6 to 8.4% of cycles, half of them "severe." The most severe form of OHSS is life threatening. Recent studies have found that donors were at less risk of OHSS when the final maturation of oocytes was induced by GnRH agonist than with recombinant hCG. Both hormones were comparable in the number of mature oocytes produced and fertilization rates.[18] [19] A larger study in the Netherlands found 10 documented cases of deaths from IVF, with a rate of 1:10,000. "All of these patients were treated with GnRH agonists and none of these cases have been published in the scientific literature." Hormone treatments that can be dangerous in the short-term may have long-term health effects.

The long-term impact of egg donation on donors has not been well studied, but apparently some evidence suggests an increased risk of ovarian cancer, and effects on fertility.[17] [20] 1 in 5 women report psychological effects from donating their eggs, both good and bad. However two-thirds women were happy with the decision to donate their eggs. The same study found that 20% of women didn't recall being aware of any physical risks.[15] Some short-term effects can be severe and the long-term effects are not well studied.

However, it appears that repetitive oocyte donation cycles does not cause accelerated ovarian aging, evidenced by absence of decreased anti-Müllerian hormone (AMH) in such women.[21]

Recipient

The recipient has a minimal risk of contracting a transmittable disease. While the donor may test negative for HIV, such testing does not exclude the possibility that the donor has contracted HIV very recently, so the recipient faces a residual risk of exposure. However, the FDA governs this and requires full infectious disease testing no more than 30 days prior to retrieval and/or transfer. Most clinics now require, however, that donors be retested a few days prior to retrieval so the risk to the recipient is minimal. Intimate partners of both the egg donor and the recipient are also tested.

The recipient also trusts that the genetic and medical history of the donor is accurate. This factor of trust should not be underestimated in importance. Donors are paid thousands of dollars; monetary compensation may attract unscrupulous individuals inclined to conceal their true motivations. However, a full psychological evaluation is required by most IVF clinics, giving an indication if the donor is trustworthy or not.

In more cases than not, there is no ongoing relationship between the donor and recipient following the cycle. Both the donor and recipient agree in formal legal documents that the donation of the eggs is final at the time of retrieval, and typically both parties would like any "relationship" to conclude at that point. Some children born from this technology will find their biological donor(s)using DNA databanks and/or registries due to secrecy and anonymity being involved.

Multiple birth is a common complication if the physician transfers too many embryos. Incidence of twin births is very high. At the present time, the ASRM clearly recommends that 1 or 2 embryos are transferred in any given cycle. (Any remaining embryos are typically frozen for future transfers.)

Custody

Generally legal documents are signed renouncing rights and responsibilities of custody on the part of the donor. Most IVF doctors will not proceed with administering medication to any donor until these documents are in place and a legal "clearance letter" confirming this understanding is provided to the doctor.

Legality

Egg donation is regulated and /or prohibited in many countries. In the United States, having an attorney draft a contract is often necessary to establish and confirm the parental rights over any child. Hiring an attorney who specializes in reproductive law is strongly recommended. Legal contracts are considered more as guidelines of intent and may be declared invalid as a child's best interest is generally considered when litigation occurs. Donor's and other participants retain their rights as well, and cannot be forced to adhere to any contract that is declared to be invalid.

The Buzzanca versus Buzzanca, 72 Cal. Rptr.2d 280 (Cal. Ct. App. 1998), established the role of the recipient, the father of the conceived child, and the child. It stated that both the recipient and the father of the child by virtue of their procreative intent, are the legal parents of the child. Therefore, the father must pay child-support even if he claims a divorce before the conception of the child.[22]

The Uniform Parentage Act (updated most recently in 2002) establishes the role of the egg recipient to the conceived child. The recipient under this act, is given complete parental responsibility of the conceived child.

Before the retrieval of the eggs from the donor, the donor must sign the Egg Donor Contract which specifies the rights of the donor with respect to the conceived child and the recipient. In this contract the donor agrees to undergo a thorough medical and psychological screening, genetic testing, and screening for communicable diseases (i.e. HIV). Also, it specifies that the egg recipient and the father of the child are the legal parents.

Donor registries

A donor registry is a registry to facilitate donor conceived people, sperm donors and egg donors to establish contact with genetic kindred. They are mostly used by donor conceived people to find genetic half-siblings from the same egg- or sperm donor.

Some donors are non-anonymous, but most are anonymous, i.e. the donor conceived person doesn't know the true identity of the donor. Still, he/she may get the donor number from the fertility clinic. If that donor had donated before, then other donor conceived people with the same donor number are thus genetic half-siblings. In short, donor registries match people who type in the same donor number.

Alternatively, if the donor number isn't available, then known donor characteristics, e.g. hair, eye and skin color may be used in matching.

Donors may also register, and therefore, donor registries may also match donors with their genetic children.

The largest registry is the Donor Sibling Registry- with more than 25,000 members, the DSR has matched almost 7,000 donor conceived people with their egg and sperm donors, as well as with their half siblings. Alternate methods of providing an information link between the donor and recipient (both agreeing to stay registered on the DSR) are often provided for in the legal document (referred to as the "Egg Donor Agreement".)

Embryo Donation

An alternative to egg donation in some couples, especially those in whom the male partner cannot provide viable sperm, is embryo donation, sometimes called "embryo adoption". Embryo donation is, as its name implies, the donation of embryos remaining after one couple's IVF treatments have been completed, to another individual or couple, followed by the placement of those embryos into the recipient woman's uterus, to facilitate pregnancy and childbirth. Embryo donation has been shown in a recent study to be more cost-effective than egg donation on a "per live birth" basis [23] . Another study has found that embryos created for one couple, using an egg donor, are often made available for donation to another couple if the first couple chooses not to use them. [24]

Psychological and social issues

Further information: Donor conceived people#Psychological and social

Common reasons to donate are to help childless couples, and, for some, the monetary compensation. Reluctance to donate may be caused by a sense of ownership and responsibility for the well-being of the offspring.[25]

Most psychological and social issues of egg donation are likely comparable to those of sperm donation.

Telling the child

Most psychologists recommend being open and honest with children from an early age. Groups for donor conceived children make a strong case for the rights of children to have access to information about their genetic background. For donor conceived children who find out after a long period of secrecy, their main grief is usually not the fact that they are not the genetic child of the couple who have raised them, but the fact that the parent or parents have kept information from or lied to them, causing loss of trust.[26] Furthermore, the overturn of the sense of who were the parents through the whole life may cause a lasting sense of imbalance and loss of control.[27]

However, there are certain circumstances where the child very likely should be told:

- When many relatives know about the donation, so that the child might find it out from somebody else.[26]
- When the recipient carries a significant genetic disease, relieving the child from fear of being a carrier.[26]
- Where the child is found to suffer from a genetically-transmitted disorder and it is necessary to take legal action which then identifies the donor.

Families sharing same donor

Having contact and meeting among families sharing the same donor generally has positive effects.[28] [29] It gives the child an extended family and helps give the child a sense of identity[29] by answering questions about the donor.[28] It is more common among *open identity*-families headed by single women.[28] Less than 1% of those seeking donor-siblings find it a negative experience, and in such cases it is mostly where the parents have disagreed with each other about how the relationship should proceed.[30]

Other family members

Grandparents of donors, often the oldest surviving progenitors, may regard the donated genetic contribution as a family asset, and may regard the donor conceived people as grandchildren.[31]

Religious Views

Some Christian leaders indicate that IVF is acceptable (but they should ensure that no fertilized embryos are discarded in the process). Many Christian couples who cannot have children thus can go for IVF, with both the husband's sperm and the wife's egg and this is in line with the church's teaching.

However the question gets trickier with donor eggs.

There are also some Christian leaders (especially Catholic) who are concerned about all in vitro fertility therapies because they disrupt the natural act of conceiving a child where gamete donations, both egg and sperm donations, are seen to "compromise the marital bond and family integrity".[32] and they encourage infertile couples to consider adoption instead.

In the Muslim Community, Sunnis are allowed fertility treatments that do not involve third parties. This rule does not allow for the donation of gametes. Shi'ite Muslims on the other hand are allowed to accept egg donations, although there are some details that prevent egg donation in some countries and regions.[33]

The permission to use an egg donor for Jewish couples is based on the decision of a rabbi, although there is no consensus in the orthodox community as to whether a child is Jewish based on the religious status of the genetic or gestational mother.[34] This distinction is important since a Jewish egg donor may be needed. This is not an issue in the reform community since only one parent, either the mother or father, must be Jewish for the child to be considered Jewish. In the orthodox community the mother must be Jewish for the child to be Jewish.

See also

- Sperm donation
- Donor conceived people

References

[1] http://www.nlm.nih.gov/cgi/mesh/2011/MB_cgi?field=uid&term=D018587

[2] Blakeslee, Sandra (1984-02-04). "Infertile Woman Has Baby Through Embryo Transfer" (http://query.nytimes.com/gst/fullpage.html?sec=health&res=9404EEDC143BF937A35751C0A962948260). *The New York Times*. . Retrieved 2009-11-05.

[3] http://www.humc.edu/calendar/careacc.html HUMC - Celebrating 50 Years of Caring

[4] Friedrich, Otto; Constable, Anne; Samghabadi, Raji (1984-09-10). "Medicine: A Legal, Moral, Social Nightmare" (http://www.time.com/time/magazine/article/0,9171,952517,00.html). *Time*. . Retrieved 2010-05-01.

[5] Wallis, Claudia (1984-09-10). "The New Origins of Life" (http://www.time.com/time/magazine/article/0,9171,952514,00.html). *TIME*. . Retrieved 2009-11-05.

[6] Friedrich, Otto; Constable, Anne; Samghabadi, Raji (1984-09-10). "Medicine: A Legal, Moral, Social Nightmare" (http://www.time.com/time/magazine/article/0,9171,952517-6,00.html). *Time*. . Retrieved 2010-05-01.

[7] http://www.obgmanagement.com/srm/pdf/first_live_birth_donation.pdf

[8] http://www.obgmanagement.com/srm.asp?id=5030

[9] *cross donor* is termed *korsdonator* in Swedish

[10] Check, JH (2002). "The shared donor oocyte program: the advantages and insights it provides in determining etiologic factors of infertility" (http://www.ccivf.com/pdf_files/pdf articles/CATEGO~6/003.PDF). *Clinical and experimental obstetrics & gynecology* **29** (4): 229–34. PMID 12635736. .

[11] Cost analysis of shared oocyte in vitro fertilization (http://www.library.nhs.uk/womenshealth/ViewResource.aspx?resID=245239) Peskin B D, Austin C, Lisbona H, Goldfarb J M. "Cost analysis of shared oocyte in vitro fertilization." *Obstetrics and Gynecology*, 1996; 88(3): 428-430

[12] Prognosis of oocyte donation cycles: a prospective comparison of the in vitro fertilization–embryo transfer cycles of recipients who used shared oocytes versus those who used altruistic donors (http://www.fertstert.org/article/S0015-0282(08)03290-1/abstract) *Fertility and Sterility*. Volume 92, Issue 3, Pages 930-936 (September 2009). Olufunso A. Oyesanya, M.D.ab, Olufemi Olufowobi, M.D.a, Wendy Ross, R.N.a, Khaldoun Sharif, M.D a, Masoud Afnan, M.D.ab

[13] https://bhed.com/pub_donor_info.php#donation Beverly Hills Egg Donation | Become an Egg Donor

[14] Egg donation (http://avapeter.com/en/egg/) Egg donor bank

[15] Kara N. Maxwell, Ina N. Cholst, Zev Rosenwaks. (2008). The incidence of both serious and minor complications in young women undergoing oocyte donation, Fertility and Sterility. 90: 2165-2171.

[16] http://pulitzercenter.org/blog/untold-stories/it%E2%80%99s-not-altruism-it%E2%80%99s-selling

[17] Textbook of Assisted Reproductive Techniques, Laboratory and Clinical Perspectives, edited by David K. Gardner, 2001

[18] Galindo, A.; Bodri, D.; Guillen, J.J.; Colodron, M.; Vernaeve, V.; Coll, O. (2009). "Triggering with HCG or GnRH agonist in GnRH antagonist treated oocyte donation cycles: a randomized clinical trial". *Gynecol Endocrinol* **25** (1): 60–6. doi:10.1080/09513590802404013. PMID 19165664.

[19] Bodri, D.; Guillen, J.J.; Galindo, A.; Mataro, D.; Pujol, A.; Coll, O. (2009). "Triggering with human chorionic gonadotropin or a gonadotropin-releasing hormone agonist gonadotropin-releasing hormone antagonist-treated oocyte donor cycles:findings of large retrospective cohort study". *Fertil Steril* **91** (2): 365–71. doi:10.1016/j.fertnstert.2007.11.049. PMID 18367175.

[20] http://health.usnews.com/articles/health/healthday/2008/12/26/risks-and-benefits-of-egg-donation-reported.html?PageNr=1
[21] Bukulmez O, Li Q, Carr BR, Leader B, Doody KM, Doody KJ (July 2009). "Repetitive oocyte donation does not decrease serum anti-Müllerian hormone levels". *Fertil. Steril.* **94** (3): 905–12. doi:10.1016/j.fertnstert.2009.05.017. PMID 19631321.
[22] http://www.law.uh.edu/healthlaw/perspectives/Reproductive/980408Child.html
[23] Finger R, Sommerfelt C, Freeman M, Wilson CK, Wade A, Daly D. A cost-effectiveness comparison of embryo donation with oocyte donation. Fertil Steril 2010;93:379-81.
[24] Hill GA, Freeman MR. Embryo disposition: Choices made by patients and donor oocyte recipients. Fertil Steril 2011;95:940-3
[25] McMahon CA, Saunders DM (November 2007). "Attitudes of couples with stored frozen embryos toward conditional embryo donation". *Fertil. Steril.* **91** (1): 140–7. doi:10.1016/j.fertnstert.2007.08.004. PMID 18053994.
[26] Donor insemination Edited by C.L.R. Barratt and I.D. Cooke. Cambridge (England): Cambridge University Press, 1993. 231 pages.
[27] A generation of sperm donor children are discovering the father they know and love is NOT their father at all. (http://www.dailymail.co.uk/femail/article-1163032/A-generation-sperm-donor-children-discovering-father-know-love-NOT-father-all.html) By Alison Smith Squire in Daily Mail. Last updated at 11:18 AM on 19th March 2009
[28] Scheib JE, Ruby A (July 2008). "Contact among families who share the same sperm donor". *Fertil. Steril.* **90** (1): 33–43. doi:10.1016/j.fertnstert.2007.05.058. PMID 18023432.
[29] T. Freeman, V. Jadva, W. Kramer, and S. Golombok. Gamete donation: parents' experiences of searching for their child's donor siblings and donor. (http://humrep.oxfordjournals.org/cgi/content/abstract/24/3/505) Human Reproduction, 2008; 24 (3): 505 DOI: 10.1093/humrep/den469
[30] Contact with donor siblings a good experience for most families (http://www.theglobeandmail.com/servlet/story/RTGAM.20090226.wldonor26/BNStory/lifeFamily/home) By HAYLEY MICK. From Thursday's Globe and Mail. February 26, 2009 at 8:58 AM EDT
[31] My scattered grandchildren (http://www.theglobeandmail.com/life/family-and-relationships/my-scattered-grandchildren/article1286201/) The Globe and Mail. Alison Motluk. Sunday, Sep. 13, 2009 07:53PM EDT
[32] http://www.albertmohler.com/commentary_read.php?cdate=2006-05-10
[33] Inhorn, M.C. 2005. IVF and gamete donation in the Muslim world. Religion and Reproductive Technologies. 46:14. http://www.aaanet.org/press/an/0502Inhorn.htm
[34] http://www.yoatzot.org/article.php?id=112

ASRM Practice Committee Reports, Fertility Sterility 82, Suppl. 1, Sept. 2004.

External links

Egg Donation (http://www.dmoz.org//Health/Reproductive_Health/Infertility/Donor_Services/Egg_Donation//) at the Open Directory Project

List_of_Mendelian_traits_in_humans

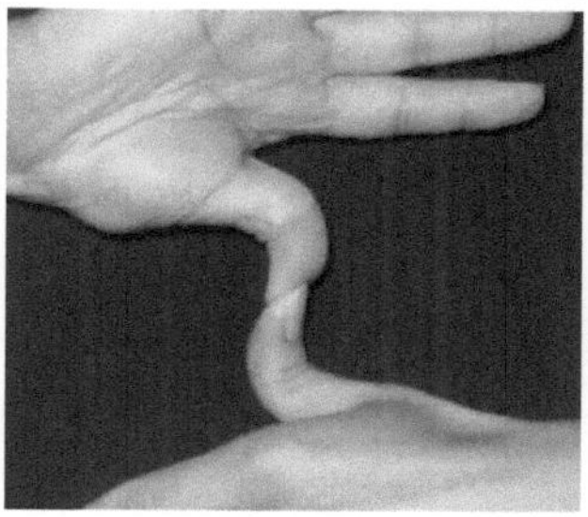

Hitchhiker's thumbs

In Mendelian inheritance, a child receiving a dominant allele from either parent will have the dominant form of the trait. Only those that received the recessive allele from both parents present with the recessive phenotype. Those that receive a dominant allele from one parent and a recessive allele from the other parent will have the dominant form of the trait. Purely Mendelian traits are a tiny minority of all traits, since most phenotypic traits exhibit incomplete dominance, codominance, and contributions from many genes.

The recessive phenotype may theoretically skip any number of generations, lying dormant in heterozygous "carrier" individuals until they have children with someone who also has the recessive allele and both pass it on to their child.

Examples

These traits include:

- Ability to taste phenylthiocarbamide (dominant)
- Ability to smell (bitter almond-like) hydrogen cyanide
- Albinism (recessive)
- Brachydactyly (shortness of fingers and toes)
- Wet (dominant) or dry (recessive) earwax
- immunity to poison ivy (dominant)
- Hitchiker's thumb (recessive)

Traits previously believed to be Mendelian

Some traits were previously believed to be Mendelian, but their inheritance is (probably) based on more complex genetic models, possibly involving more than one gene. These include [1] :

- Eyecolor
- Hair color
- Morton's toe
- Tongue rolling
- Widow's peak (allele)
- Detached (dominant) or attached (recessive) earlobes

See also

- Heritability
- Human genetic variation
- Human genetic clustering

References

[1] http://udel.edu/~mcdonald/mythintro.html

External links

- OMIM Online Mendelian Inheritance in Man (http://www.ncbi.nlm.nih.gov/omim)

Earlobe

Earlobe

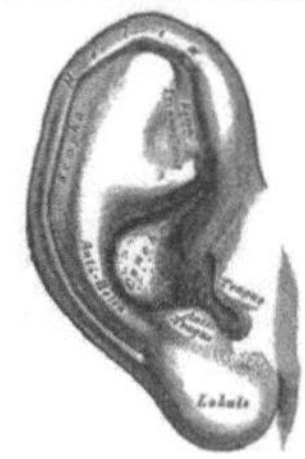

Latin	*lobulus auriculae (singular), lobuli auricularum (plural)*
Gray's	*subject #229 1034* [1]
System	Auditory system

The **human earlobe** is composed of tough areolar and adipose connective tissues, lacking the firmness and elasticity of the rest of the pinna. Since the earlobe does not contain cartilage it has a large blood supply and may help to warm the ears and maintain balance. However earlobes are not generally considered to have any major biological function.[2] The earlobe contains many nerve endings, and for some people is an erogenous zone.

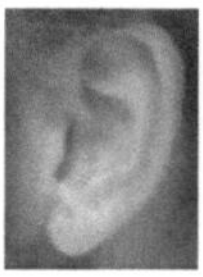

A free earlobe

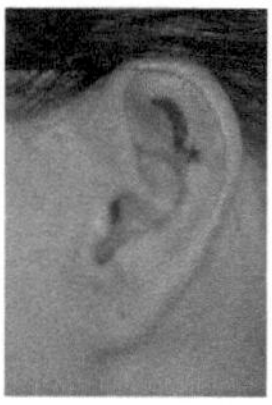

An attached earlobe, with piercing and tattoo

Size and shape

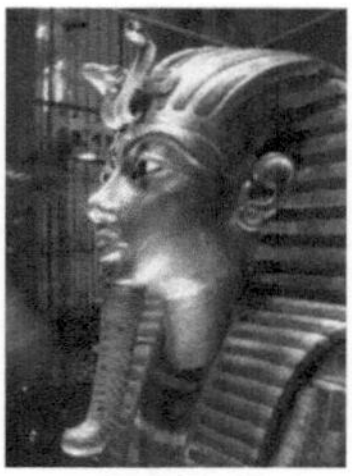

Tutankhamen displaying a stretched earlobe piercing.

Earlobes average about 2 cm long, and elongate slightly with age.[3] Although the "free" vs. "attached" appearance of earlobes is often presented as an example of a simple "one gene - two alleles" Mendelian trait in humans, several studies suggest that the story is not that simple.[4] [5] A quick survey of your friends will reveal that earlobes do not all fall neatly into either the "free" or the "attached" categories; there is a continuous range from one extreme to the other, suggesting the influence of several genes.

Earlobes are normally smooth, but occasionally exhibit creases. Creased earlobes are sometimes associated with genetic disorders in children, including Beckwith-Wiedemann syndrome.[6] In some early studies, earlobe creases were alleged to be associated with an increased risk of heart attack and coronary heart disease; however, more recent studies have concluded that since earlobes become more creased with age, and older people are more likely to experience heart disease than younger people, age may account for the findings linking heart attack to earlobe creases.[6] The earlobe crease is also called Frank's Sign.

Earlobe piercing

Around the world and throughout human history, the earlobe is the most common location for a body piercing. It is common to tear the earlobe with the weight of very heavy earring, or a traumatic pull of an earring. Some cultures practice earlobe stretching, using piercing ornaments to stretch and enlarge the earlobes. Sailors used to believe that piercing one earlobe gave greater acuity in the opposite ear.

References

[1] http://education.yahoo.com/reference/gray/subjects/subject?id=229#p1034

[2] Popelka, Gerald (August 31, 1999). "Re: Why do we have earlobes, what are they for, since when?" (http://www.madsci.org/posts/archives/aug99/934627537.Ev.r.html). MadSci Network. .

[3] Azaria R, Adler N, Silfen R, Regev D, Hauben DJ (June 2003). "Morphometry of the adult human earlobe: a study of 547 subjects and clinical application" (http://meta.wkhealth.com/pt/pt-core/template-journal/lwwgateway/media/landingpage.htm?issn=0032-1052&volume=111&issue=7&spage=2398). *Plast. Reconstr. Surg.* **111** (7): 2398–402; discussion 2403–4. doi:10.1097/01.PRS.0000060995.99380.DE. PMID 12794488. .

[4] Lai LY, Walsh RJ (1966). "Observations on ear lobe types". *Acta Genet Stat Med* **16** (3): 250–7. PMID 5953713.

[5] Dutta, P, Ganguly, P (1965). "Further observations on ear lobe attachment". *Acta Genet Statist Med* **15**: 77–86. PMID 14277139.

[6] "" (http://www.nlm.nih.gov/medlineplus/ency/article/003045.htm). . Retrieved March 17, 2012. Medline Plus, a service of the U.S. National Library of Medicine, National Institutes of Health: "Some studies have found that people with earlobe creases have a greater risk for heart attack than others. More recent research suggests that earlobe creases are more common in older people, and that age, not the presence of creases, accounts for the increased heart attack risk."

Article Sources and Contributors

Parent *Source*: http://en.wikipedia.org/w/index.php?title=Parent *Contributors*: 16@r, 5dollabill, Aaron Kauppi, Absopositutely, Academic Challenger, Admiral06, Ahoerstemeier, Alansohn, AlexyGalaxy, AllPurposeGamer, Allens, American Samurai, Ancheta Wis, Angie Y., AnonGuy, Antonio Lopez, Anubhavk1980, Arakunem, Arjun01, Arnon Chaffin, Azumanga1, Babajazz!, Bbetsy, Beetstra, Bennetto, Bibliomaniac15, Bkkbrad, Blotto adrift, Bobo192, Boing! said Zebedee, Bongwarrior, Brandmeister, Bussys, Butko, CIreland, COMPFUNK2, Calliopejen1, Calvin 1998, Can't sleep, clown will eat me, Charles Matthews, Chris the speller, Ciderbarrel, Ckatz, Click23, Closedmouth, Codetiger, CommonsDelinker, Courcelles, Cubs Fan, Cuddlybunnybecki, Cyberman101, DUFFFMANN, Dadtalkuz, Daveenvoy, Ddcc, Dekisugi, Deli nk, Demmy, Destinero, Dillard421, Discospinster, Dlattari96, Dragix, DragonflySixtyseven, Drunkenmoron95, Dspradau, Durova, Eliz81, Epbr123, Excirial, Ezeu, Fences and windows, Ferengi, Fieldday-sunday, FisherQueen, Flauto Dolce, Fratrep, FreplySpang, Fyyer, Gail, Gdje je nestala duša svijeta, Geoff Plourde, Georgia guy, Ginsengbomb, Gogo Dodo, Gracezen, Guess123456789101112, HamburgerRadio, Helicoptor, Howsa12, Hwlleeo, IRP, Icestorm815, IvyHeath, J.delanoy, JASpencer, JavierMC, Jimothytrotter, Jincy32, Johnuniq, Jojit fb, Jonemerson, Jordanstrm, Jusdafax, KGasso, Kerowren, Kevinkor2, Khalid Mahmood, KillerChihuahua, Kingrattus, Kukkurovaca, Lethe, Lotje, M phillips58?, MER-C, MacsBug, Macy, Mark Arsten, Mark91, Masnevets, Materialscientist, Matlefebvre20, Merope, Mikaey, Moink, Momo san, Montrealais, Mr Adequate, Mr Stephen, MrOllie, Mucus, N1RK4UDSK714, N5iln, Nakon, NathanoNL, NellieBly, NeutriceH5, Nickvailas10, Nivix, Ohnoitsjamie, Olegwiki, Orangemike, Oxymoron83, PTime, ParentPages, Parentline, Pedro, Peko, Penbat, Phaedriel, Pharaoh of the Wizards, Pharcshad, Phearson, Philip Trueman, Piggepang, PleaseStand, Poobread, Portalian, QDJones, Raso mk, Red dwarf, RekishiEJ, Retama, Rhrad, Richard001, RingtailedFox, Rixs, S19991002, SD5, STGM, Sant008, SchuminWeb, Scrumpet, Seb opie, Serein (renamed because of SUL), Severa, Sk8rlove13, Slakr, Smurphy456, Sonic3KMaster, Spiritualism, Stef554true, TJRC, Tayste, The Man in Question, The Thing That Should Not Be, Tijfo098, Tinton5, Tpb, Tregoweth, Tvrocks267, UNIT A4B1, Ulric1313, Unschool, Usgnus, Versus22, Vicenarian, Violask81976, Vliegen, Voortle, WadeSimMiser, WikHead, Wikipelli, Willking1979, Wrad, Wykis, X42bn6, Zargulon, Zdub723, Ziaia, Zodon, 263 anonymous edits

Offspring *Source*: http://en.wikipedia.org/w/index.php?title=Offspring *Contributors*: Aaron Kauppi, Alberto Orlandini, Altenmann, Anythingyouwant, Azertus, BD2412, Bart133, Bonalaw, Bookandcoffee, Btyner, Can't sleep, clown will eat me, Dark Lord of the Sith, Delta Tango, Doctorfluffy, ENeville, Elf, Esanchez7587, Fangusu, Firetrap9254, Galoubet, Gilliam, Ginkgo100, Hede2000, Herostratus, Humbabba, Icarus3, Idns310, Idonotlikepeas, InShaneee, Jaxson666, Jeronimo, Jessicagirls, Jigen III, Jon Stockton, KGasso, Kalaiarasy, Keivan.f, MBFMETAL, Marcus Qwertyus, Metalmasta5, Milant, Montrealais, Nono64, Oxymoron83, Paxsimius, Penbat, Petiatil, Petrb, Phluid61, Plrk, Putnum, QuackOfaThousandSuns, Quintote, R'n'B, Richard001, Rillian, Rjd0060, Robertmh, Saukkomies, Sexygirl2, Shadoks, Shanes, Smoky Mc Weed, Soumyasch, Spittlespat, SunnySideOfStreet, Superbeecat, Tchonch, The Man in Question, Uncle Milty, Visor, Von Karma, William Avery, Wolfgang1018, Yowuza, 93 anonymous edits

Ancestor *Source*: http://en.wikipedia.org/w/index.php?title=Ancestor *Contributors*: 7ofWiMe, Acroterion, Alansohn, Animum, Asarlaí, Astronautics, Azoreg, BD2412, BMF81, Black Kite, CBM, Cadsuane Melaidhrin, CanisRufus, Chelsea99, Cribbswh, Crzrussian, DIEGO RICARDO, David Little, Dbachmann, DeltaRhoPhi, Dialectric, Discospinster, Download, Ehrenkater, Epf, Firien, Galoubet, Gershwinrb, Grutness, Haljolad, HenryLi, Henrygb, Ihcoyc, Ike9898, Isnow, Isomorphic, Isotope23, JWB, Jackbrown, Jayjg, Jjron, JohnAlbertRigali, Jojit fb, Karada, Kelly Martin, Kelvin125, Kjramesh, Knowledge for All, Koterpillar, Lahiru k, Lenoxus, MALLUS, MNRoss, Manway, Mathias-S, Mayooranathan, MidnightBlueMan, Mkill, Modest Genius, Monkeyboy2000, Morwen, Mr.crabby, Neo-Jay, Nick123, Oda Mari, OrthodoxLinguist, Otchster, Pavel Vozenilek, Peak, Pearle, Penbat, Phantomsteve, Philip Trueman, PhilipO, Rich Farmbrough, Ringbang, Romanm, Rumping, Scottsigler, Scwlong, Solipsist, Steveprutz, T@nn, TJ Dizzle, Thaurisil, The Man in Question, The Ogre, Thecup, Tokyogirl79, Vmrgrsergr, Vrenator, Wayiran, Wmahan, Woer$, XXxChrisrawr, Yunshui, ZeroGiga, דוד55, 101 anonymous edits

Generation *Source*: http://en.wikipedia.org/w/index.php?title=Generation *Contributors*: 1800Allen, 21st century Susan, Aaronsav, Adamantios, Adjeadja, Ale jrb, Alvalleygrl, Alyeska, Amake, Androo123, Angr, Another Believer, Arthena, Arthur Rubin, Azoreg, Babbler, Badanedwa, Barek, BatteryIncluded, Ben James Ben, Benw, Bezymov, Biker Biker, Bill, Bill.martin, Bjoh249, Blairius, Bluemoose, Bobo192, Brianmacian, Brunton, Buckosucko212, CTSCo, CatJar, CaveatLector, Ccacsmss, Ccrowe1990, Cgingold, Chickenandchhorn, ChikeJ, Chuunen Baka, Clevercat17, ColdFusion650, Corenabh, Coreyloum, CosineKitty, CreativeSoul7981, Ctachme, Cyan, DBigXray, DLBY, David Vincents, Davidsonj, Dekisugi, Dennis Brown, Der Falke, Deville, Devon t, Dgcaskey, Diceman, Diego Grez, DocWatson42, Dr kayoz, Dylan Lake, ERhaught, Edward321, Eep², Ej926, El0i, Emily Wolfinger, Eminemshow123, Epbr123, Ephemeral Insanity, Extreme gnarliness, Fabartus, Facts707, Falcon8765, Fastily, Fear and loathing, Fifo, Fingers-of-Pyrex, Fluffernutter, Fr33kman, Freechild, Fufu4u, Funandtrvl, Fyrael, G.Tenzing, Getphysical68, Gpietsch, Gtrmp, Guessing Game, Hairy Dude, Hephaestos, Hertz1888, Hmains, Hmusseau, Im4earth, Indon, Infrogmation, IstvanWolf, J.delanoy, JForget, JHunterJ, JaGa, JackDayton, Jacthelad, JakeVortex, Jason Fitz, Jatkins, Jeff G., Joseph Solis in Australia, Joshdboz, Jumping cheese, Jusjih, K.d.stauffer, Katydidit, KimvdLinde, Kinema, King Semsem, Koakhtzvigad, Krich, Kyng, La goutte de pluie, Ledboots, Letowskie, LilHelpa, Lilac Soul, Limsont, Lipothymia, Lord Loxley, Lradrama, Malik Shabazz, MarSch, Markhurd, Martarius, Mayur, Mickeyp2814, Mistress Selina Kyle, Mithent, Mshara1, Msirois, Mydogategodshat, Mytildebang, NHJG2, Nasa-verve, NawlinWiki, NeilN, NeonMerlin, Newfraferz87, Nick Number, Nickg, Nightkey, ONEder Boy, OldakQuill, OliviaKoenig, Osarius, Park3r, Patmaher, Patty Lester, Peregrine981, Phil Bridger, PhnomPencil, Piecraft, Poco a poco, Polgárj, Portia327, Puchiko, R'n'B, Reddi, Reenad84, Rich Farmbrough, Rjwilmsi, RobertMfromLI, Rothskin, RoyBoy, Rudykog, SGGH, Sandberry, Sandstein, Sarah, Sarcha 45, Scriberius, Sgore, Shadowblade, Shamak, Smilo Don, Sonicyouth86, Spiffy sperry, SpikeZOM, SpringSloth, Spy007au, Startswithj, Steel, Stephaniesoftball, Steven Walling, Stevenmitchell, Stevertigo, Strundle, Supt. of Printing, TOttenville8, Tabletop, TaintedMustard, Tarheel95, Tdankmyer, The Man in Question, The Obento Musubi, TheCustomOfLife, Thebigjefferson, Theflyer, Thetrickster69, Thewebb, Thingg, Thoglette, Tide rolls, Tillwe, Tinlinkin, TreadingWater, Treisijs, True Pagan Warrior, Tuba59, Tyler, Unitanode, UnqstnableTruth, V1oletv, Valfontis, Vman89, WLU, Walter Görlitz, Wapondaponda, WikiDao, Wiwaxia, Woohookitty, YUL89YYZ, Yamamoto Ichiro, Yamara, Zanter, 479 anonymous edits

Birth *Source*: http://en.wikipedia.org/w/index.php?title=Birth *Contributors*: *drew, 16@r, 2004-12-29T22:45Z, 7, Aaron Kauppi, Ace Oliveira, Addshore, AgentPeppermint, Ahoerstemeier, Akaohio, Alan Liefting, Alansohn, Aldio Yudha Trisandy, Alicelight, Allstarecho, AmyNelson, Animonster, Antonio Lopez, Argon233, ArielGold, Artisol2345, Ashley Y, Backtable, Barbara Shack, Bcatt, Beaumont, Beland, Bidgee, BillShurts, Billinghurst, Blackshadow1998, Bobo192, Bongwarrior, Booyabazooka, BovineBeast, Bumdarts, C+C, COMPFUNK2, Can't sleep, clown will eat me, Captain-tucker, Celique, Chacha8, Chaojoker, Cheezeman, Ckatz, Cobi, Commander Keane, ConCompS, Coredesat, Courcelles, Crickeys, Cuddlyable3, DanP, Delldot, Denkealsobin, DerHexer, Diciassettedimaggio, Ding, Djhills, Dlohcierekim, Donniebravo, Dougweller, Drmies, Essjay, Evercat, Ewlyahoocom, Faustnh, Fennec, FieryTurdGymnast, Flyguy649, Frally123, Fratrep, Fretwurst, Fwgoebel, Geoharee, Geniac, Gillyweed, Ginkgo100, Gogo Dodo, Graham87, Gscshoyru, HAL(Old), HalJor, Hammerdickulous, Harryboyles, Hdt83, Hede2000, Heeheehahahohoho, HexaChord, Husond, Hut 8.5, IW.HG, Iamaloser12, Ilovericky, IndulgentReader, IngerAlHaosului, Jambornik, JamesBWatson, Jameshfisher, Jay, JennyMHatch, Jkhbgcdijkhbnomkj, John of Reading, Joie de Vivre, Joost 99, Juliepatt, Jusdafax, KellyPhD, Knutux, Kukini, L Kensington, LEHarth, Lima, LittleOldMe, Lotje, Lyrl, Mac, Mad Max, Madaise, Madhero88, Magister Mathematicae, MarkSutton, Masrudin, Mateuse71, Maustrauser, Max Duchess, Medicobaby, Michael Hardy, Mickihirsch, Mojska, Montrealais, Moreschi, Multixfer, Müslimix, Nadinemaina, Nandesuka, NawlinWiki, Nevit, Nigholith, NinjaCharlie, NoLightofMyOwn, Nsusa, NuclearWinner, Nyttend backup, OOODDD, Ohjung5000, Olegwiki, Owen, Pablodiego15, Pattych, Pax6, Persian Poet Gal, Philip Trueman, Philippe, Pilotguy, Pizzatime, Quantumobserver, Quixada, Qupqugiak, R'n'B, RainbowOfLight, Rajkiandris, Ranveig, Rje, Robert Bond, Rossami, Roxie09, Rrmadore, Ryulong, SD6-Agent, SOK, Sagaciousuk, Samw, Sandy sakura, Sannse, Secretlondon, Seraphim, Seth Ilys, Severa, Shadowjams, ShakataGaNai, Shawn fard, ShelfSkewed, SlackerMom, Sly-eye, Soumyasch, Stevertigo, Superjustinbros., Symane, Ta bu shi da yu, Taggard, Tarquin, Tbhotch, Template namespace initialisation script, The Anome, The Obento Musubi, The Rambling Man, Thedjatclubrock, Thegonugget, Thewayforward, Thingg, Tide rolls, Tim Berkey, Tom Morris, Tombomp, Tythepi, Tznkai, Una Smith, V.narsikar, Valkrie1496, Vancouver Outlaw, WLU, Waggers, Warbirdadmiral, Wayiran, Wikipelli, Wisdom89, Xdamr, Yachtsman1, Yamamoto Ichiro, Ychastnik APL, Yoninah, ZooFari, Zzuuzz, 235 anonymous edits

Interpersonal_relationship *Source*: http://en.wikipedia.org/w/index.php?title=Interpersonal_relationship *Contributors*: 16@r, 2D, Aaron Brenneman, Aaron Kauppi, AbsolutDan, Acidburn24m, AdamZMann, Addshore, Aduialion, Alansohn, Alephh, Allmethods, Allmightyduck, Ancheta Wis, Andrew Gray, AndyTheGrump, Andycjp, Angela, Animequalslife, Arno Matthias, Arthena, B, BMF81, Barek, Beginning, Beland, Benjiboi, Blackjack676, Bobbyd1234, Bonás, Brandon.macuser, CJ, CQ, Cachola316, CambridgeBayWeather, Capricorn42, Cgingold, CieloEstrellado, Civil Engineer III, Cncs wikipedia, Cohesion, Courcelles, Cuaxdon, Cumbiadude, DARTH SIDIOUS 2, DBigXray, DMacks, Da baum, Deborah909, Delicious carbuncle, DerHexer, Dieter Simon, Discospinster, Dmitri Lytov, Dmoss, DocWatson42, DoctorW, Dominicguadiz, DorisH, Download, Drboisclair, Drdac, Dsmith113093, ERcheck, EagleFan, Ec5618, Eekerz, Eequor, El C, Eleuther, Emilyken, Erianna, Ermeyers, Ewawer, Extransit, Ezeu, Favonian, Fenice, FiP, Finavon, Firien, Focus, Fredrik, Fryed-peach, Funandtrvl, Future Perfect at Sunrise, Galoubet, Ginsengbomb, Gioto, Glenn, Gmeader3, Goblin Prince, Gogo Dodo, Gpwhld, GreatAlfredini, Gwernol, Hadal, Haiduc, Happyritzo, Happysailor, Hello cello, Homerjay, II MusLiM HyBRiD II, Ilstruzzo, InNotOf3e5, Indon, Interloper2, Iridescent, It Is Me Here, Ixfd64, J.delanoy, JJJJust, JaGa, Javert, Jcbutler, Jcidado, Jedigiorgio, Jeff3000, Jeffrey Mall, Jidanni, Jimphilos, JohnC, Johnkarp, Joie de Vivre, Jojalozzo, Jojit fb, Jonathan.s.kt, Jonelee223, Jrgetsin, Jtneill, Judgesurreal777, Juliancolton, Kahar5, Karada, Kc62301, Keilana, Kiko4564, Kilo-Lima, Kozuch, Kraybilr, Kukini, Kuratipas, KuroiShiroi, KyraVixen, Lacrimosus, Ladokhau, Latka, Lauradimmock, Levineps, Lilbow3, Little guru, Lotje, Lova Falk, Lradrama, Luna Santin, Lunchscale, Madame Sosostris, Maratanos, Marc Venot, Matty3672, Maunus, Maury Markowitz, McGeddon, McSly, MediaMangler, Melanie27, Menchi, Merlion444, MethaneSymphony, Michael Hardy, Michael93555, Midas touch, Mihi502, Mike Rosoft, MilitaryTarget, Mlpearc, MovingTree, Mr. Absurd, Mr. Billion, MrOllie, Muffuletta, Nadyes, Ndenison, Neddyseagoon, Neitherday, Next Paige, Nick, Norafem, ONEder Boy, Oldlaptop321, Orange Suede Sofa, PL290, PSY7, Pais, Patrick, Pearle, Pedant17, Penbat, Petersam, PhnomPencil, Piotrus, Planefreak25, Poor Yorick, Prasadevrk, Pretzelpaws, Prolog, Psantora, Quadell, RandomP, Raysecurity, Rbj, Reaper Eternal, RedWordSmith, Rfc1394, Rhazs, Rich257, Richardsonkt, Robert Merkel, Rockfang, Rodasmith, Ronz, Rosaline lin, Rsabbatini, Rurp, SJP, Sadi Carnot, Sanya3, Sarrus, Sars, Scott Burley, ScottPetullo, Seanmcclatchey, Sheriroserocks, Sietse Snel, Simesa, Simon Kilpin, SimonP, SirGrant, Skakkle, Slakr, Smcg8374, Snowolf, SoCalSuperEagle, SofiaManteria, Soulmater, Soulwork, Special-T, Staeiou, Stay, SteinbDJ, Supintor19will, Susfele, Svaryk, Tagishsimon, TakuyaMurata, Tarheel 54, Tccr100, The Transhumanist, The Transhumanist (AWB), The Ukearchy, Theologianguy, Tide rolls, Tim Starling, Tommyjb, Tsuchiya Hikaru, UchihaDaisy, Uncle Milty, Vanished user 39948282, Velella, Viriditas, Vsmith, Walsha13, Wavesmikey, Weathermandan, Wikid77, Winchelsea, Woohookitty, Yahgoo, Yeoview, Zhou Yu, Ziji, Zondor, Zzuuzz, 359 anonymous edits

Gene *Source*: http://en.wikipedia.org/w/index.php?title=Gene *Contributors*: -), 162.129.26.xxx, 168..., 2ndAccount, 96well, Abductive, Abe5red, Access Denied, Acebulf, Acegikmo1, Achero, Achowat, AdamRetchless, Addshore, AdjustShift, Afasmit, Agathman, AgentPeppermint, Ahoerstemeier, Aitias, Akradecki, Aksttt, Alansohn, Alex.tan, Aliciaa90099, AlphaEta, Aminoacid91, Amorymeltzer, Anaxial, Andallo, Andonic, Andrea105, Andrewbadr, Andrewjlockley, Andycjp, Antandrus, Anthere, Antonov86, Archer3, Arendedwinter, Asha Vaughn, AstarothCY, Athf1234, Atulsnischal, Avoided, AxelBoldt, Ayla, Bachrach44, Badseed, Basement12, Battyofiron03, Bender235, Bernard10124, Bevo, Blah696969, Blanchardb, Bobblewik, Bobo192, Bogey97, Bongwarrior, Bozzo07, Brian0918, Brunton, Bryan Derksen, C'est moi, Can't sleep, clown will eat me, CanisRufus, Capim Dourado, Capricorn42, CatherineMunro, Cbailey7, CesarB, Ceyockey, Chameleon, Chaos, Chihuahuau, Chillllls, Chriff, CinnamonITFC, Ciphers, Cjamesh507, Classcutie7, Claviclehorn, Clicketyclack, ClockworkSoul, Cnsnmrt, Cody5, Coffee, Cohesion, ColinFine, Colonies Chris, Cometstyles, Computerjoe, ConfuciusOrnis, Conversion script, Courcelles, Craigy144, Cunya, Cureden, Curiouscorey, Cuvtixo, Cyberevil, Cyberstrike2000x, DARTH SIDIOUS 2, DBooth, DMacks, DVD R W, Dark Tichondrias, Davemck, David Gerard, David Shear, Dawnseeker2000, DeadEyeArrow, DeadlyAssassin, Denisarona, DerHexer, Discospinster, Dlohcierekim, DoctorDNA, Dogcow, Dogface, Donkeylove123, Dpen2000, Dr.Kilioth, Drphilharmonic, Dufresne77, Duncharris, Dysprosia, Echuck215, Edmund Gordon Gey, Edward Gordon Gey, Edwardlai1992, Egmontaz, Ehamberg, Elassint, Eleassar, Electricsforlife, Eloquence, ElspethB, EmersonLowry, Emilyrader, Emolovekills, Epbr123, Eric Forste, Eszett, Ettrig, Etxrge, Ewawer, Excirial, Explicit, Felizdenovo, Fieldday-sunday, Filll, Flewis, Floppy the bunnyx, Florentino floro, Flyleaflaceymosley, Fnielsen, Forluvoft, Francisco Cardenas, Francs2000, Frangibility, Fred Bradstadt, Fred Hsu, FredMcGary, FreplySpang, Func, Fvw, G3pro, GLHamilton, Galoubet, Gary King, Gell0065, Gene Ward Smith, Genetics411, Geno-Supremo, GetAgrippa, Ggrimes, Giftlite, Gilliam, Giugiu427, Gjuggler, Go Me Go, Gogo Dodo, Gomackay, Gomm, Goodtoknowbob, Graft, GrahamColm, GrayFullbuster, Guettarda, Gujulla.rahul, Gulmammad, Gwernol, Gyll, Hadal, Haham hanuka, HalJor, HamburgerRadio, Harvestgalaxy, Hazelgrace07, Helloarnold, Hellogorge10, Heron, Herostratus, HexaChord, Hilario w, Historystudent122, IRP, Iamaboy123, Ifetobi17, Incecosa, Indon, Inter, Iridescent, IstvanWolf, Ivan T., Ivo, J.delanoy, JD554, JDG, JPLeRouzic, JWSchmidt, Ja 62, Jackrm, Jaguarlaser, Jakob Suckale, JamesHilt62, JamesMLane, Jauerback, Jauhienij, Jay Litman, Jbray3179, Jebus989, Jeffrey O. Gustafson, Jerryseinfeld, Jessemv, Jesshay, Jfdwolff, JimVC3, Jimmy Pitt, Jlc123456789, Jmnbatista, Joconnol, John Fader, John of Reading, John11711, JohnArmagh, JohnJohn, Johnraciti, Johnuniq, JonHarder, Jonathanstray, Joymmart, Jrugordon, Ju66l3r, Jusjih, Jwissick, Jytdog, KGasso, Kaeleto, Karenjc, Karlbrezner, Katalaveno, Kbradnam, Ke4roh, Keesiewonder, Kierano, Killiondude, KimvdLinde, Kineticpro, King of Hearts, Kku, Kswilson, Kukini, Kurykh, Kyle Barbour, Kzollman, Lam Kin Keung, Lantonov, Larouxp12, Larsobrien, Latka, Lear's Fool, LeaveSleaves, LedgendGamer, Lee, Lee Daniel Crocker, Lexor, Lfh, Lightmouse, Lightofglory, Lil brooksy, Lilied1, LinDrug, Llywrch, Longhair, Looxix, Lotje, Luepke, Luna Santin, Luuva, MER-C, ML5, MPerel, Madeleine Price Ball, Magnus Manske, Mai-tai-guy, Major Despard, Makwy2, MarcoTolo, Marek69, Marj Tiefert, Mark Renier, MarkS, MarvintheParanoidAndroid, Masterofsuspense, Masterpiece2000, Matdrodes, Materialscientist, Mav, McDogm, Mcrosenstein, Memestream, Merube 89, MetsFan76, Mgiganteus1, Mh40, Michael Devore, Michael Greiner, Michael Hardy, Micheb, Miguel Andrade, Mikael Häggström, Mike2vil, Mikeo, Mikker, Million Moments, Millmoss, MinaFam, Minimac, Mohrflies, Moink, Moppatop, Mordgier, Mrdice, Mschel, Murtasa, Mustbcrackers, Mwanner, Mxn, Mycophage, Mygerardromance, NBeale, NCurse, NHRHS2010, Namazu-tron, Narayanese, Natalie Erin, NawlinWiki, Neelix, Neoprote, NerdyScienceDude, Neutrality, Nickayy77, NicolasAzurrrie, Nivix, Nnemo, Noctibus, Number 04, Nuno Tavares, Oda Mari, Oliver Pereira, Onco p53, Opabinia regalis, Ospalh, OwenX, Oxymoron83, PFHLai, PL290, Palnu, Para, Pascal.Tesson, Pathh, Pax:Vobiscum, Pcarbonn, Pearle, Pekaje, Persian Poet Gal, Pgan002, Pharaoh of the Wizards, Phil Boswell, Philip Trueman, PhnomPencil, Physicistjedi, Piano non troppo, Pinethicket, Pjvpjv, Plasticman83, Plastikspork, Pmj, Ponder, Proquence, Psychodolly, Ptr123, Pvosta, Pwb, Pádraic MacUidhir, Qertis, QuiteUnusual, Quizkajer, Qutezuce, RG2, RMHED, Rabid Lemur, RadioFan, Ragesoss, Ranveig, Raul654, RazorICE, Razorflame, Reach Out to the Truth, Reaper Eternal, RedWolf, Redrose64, Res2216firestar, Revilonnud, Rholton, Rhombus, Rich Farmbrough, Richard Taylor, Richard001, Rico12121212, Rikuansem13, Rjwilmsi, Rob Hooft, Roland Deschain, Romanm, Ronhjones, Rpeh, SS2005, Sam Hocevar, Samsara, Saravask, Satori Son, Saturnight, Sayeth, SchfiftyThree, Sciurinæ, Scottman07, Scottveirs, Scratlikesacorns, Seraphim, Serinde, Serkewt, Setanta747 (locked), Sgb235, Shadowjams, Shawnhath, Shenme, Shizhao, Shyamal, Siddhant, Sigmalmtd, Silivrenion, SimonP, Singularitarian, Sionus, Sjakkalle, Sjjupadhyay, Skater, Skizzik, Slon02, Slrubenstein, Sluzzelin, Smartse, Smb1001, Snow storm in Eastern Asia, Snowolf, Snoyes, Sodium, Sole Soul, Somdna, Sonett72, Sophus Bie, Steel, Stefanomione, Steinsky, SteveChervitzTrutane, Sting au, Stuhacking, Suffusion of Yellow, Sundar, SuperG2daMAX, Suriel1981, Suspekt, Susurrus, Susvolans, Sverdrup, Svick, Sweikart, Szajci, TakuyaMurata, Tarotcards, Taw, Taxman, Tczscion, Tekkaman, Test100000, Test19791979, Tharanii17, Thatguyflint, The Anome, The Evil Spartan, The High Fin Sperm Whale, The Thing That Should Not Be, The wub, TheSuave, Thecheesykid, Thehelpfulone, Think outside the box, Thunderbird2, Tickopa, Tide rolls, Tigerghost, Tim bates, TimVickers, Tito4000, Tmh, Tobby72, Tokenhost, Tom Morris, Tosendo, TransControl, Trekphiler, Trevor DE, Trevoreno, Tsanth, Tweek49, Uncle Dick, UtherSRG, Vanished user, Versus22, Vh6666, WJetChao, Waldow, Wannapwray, Wavelength, Weyes, WhaleyTim, Wikiborg, Wikieditor06, Wikipelli, Wilke, Williamb, WillowW, Wilson44691, Wise Sage150, Wj32, Wknight94, Wmahan, Wolfrock, Wombatcat, Woogee, Woohookitty, Wrt, Wwwwzzzz, Xaxafrad, Xiner, Xlonlonx, Xrmach, Yashgaroth, Yidisheryid, You wouldnt dare block me., Youandme, Yourmomssmalldick, Youssefsan, Ytrottier, Yurik, Zarius, Zashaw, 1095 anonymous edits

Foster_care *Source*: http://en.wikipedia.org/w/index.php?title=Foster_care *Contributors*: (jarbarf), 2over0, 7mike5000, 90, A More Perfect Onion, AWeidman, Addshore, Adoptwatchdog, Afterfostercare, AgentPeppermint, Ale jrb, Alexnathanson, Alpha Quadrant, Altenmann, Andycjp, Anoldtreeok, Atchom, Auntof6, Awbeal, Bachcell, Battat, Beetstra public, Betacommand, Bloebig, Blownfire, Bobo192, Bongoramsey, BrainyBabe, Brandon.macuser, BrendanAdkins, Brideshead, Brilliant Pebble, Brona, Brossow, Buddhafinder, Bussys, Calgary, CarbonCopy, Catgut, Ccacsmss, CelticLabyrinth, Cgingold, Chickeyd, Chinamentalhealth, Chris the speller, Chuckster2.0, Cloverweave, Cmdrjameson, Cookiedog, Corvus cornix, Courtney1408, CustardJack, Cvos, DARTH SIDIOUS 2, DPeterson, DVD R W, Darklilac, Dasani, Deadgnome, Dennisseger, DerHexer, Discospinster, Dmlandfair, Docu, Download, Edderso, Egil, El C, Ellsworth, English102lala, EoGuy, Epbr123, Eric-Wester, Erikjmartin, Esthertaffet, FClef, FF2010, Factfinder42, Factual tom, Fainites, Fayenatic london, Fellie9, FisherQueen, Flowanda, Fostercarealum, Fostercarevic, Fosterclub, Fosterparentcollege, Frankie0607, Freechild, GB fan, Gaius Cornelius, GeneLesterisaMan, Gothbag, Graham87, Grutness, Guy Peters, Halmstad, Harryeds, Headbomb, Hmrox, Huon, Hysteria18, Ikzing, Imapwnu, Inclusivedisjunction, Innab, Ira01, Iridescent, Ixfd64, JAn Dudík, JForget, JHunterJ, Jackmiami, Jakrieger, Japanbasedpsychologist, Jefiner, Jevansen, Jim Douglas, John of Reading, JohnChrysostom, Jordanstoltz, Journey73, Jpeeling, Jredmond, Juhy27, Juliancolton, JustAGal, K keith, Kartano, Kidlittle, Kilom691, Kjkolb, Knox2007, Kvlesher, Larensegal, Leaabc123, Lelek310, Leslie Mateus, Leviel, Licon, Lindentree, Ling.Nut, Littleboy58, LokiClock, Lova Falk, Lyc. cooperi, MJ94, Macosnine, Maelbrigda, Mallignamius, Martarius, Materialscientist, Mauls, Me4him, MehStrongBadMeh, Merope, Midwestsmith, Minasirkin, Mlandi11, Moeron, Mono, Msr69er, Muhandes, Mygerardromance, NOTLWolfie, NawlinWiki, Neverquick, Nordicviking, Nspehar08, Odie5533, Oxymoron83, P.powers2, PATH Foster Homes, Pablobenja, Pakaran, Palmcluster, Parsla, Paul Knowlton, Penbat, Peppedeninno, PigFlu Oink, Pinethicket, Pmlineditor, Poelcq, Pro Reality, Ps07swt, Pseudomyrmex, Quarl, QuiteUnusual, RJFJR, Raidon Kane, RalphLender, Redsox04, Renaissancee, Risingstar12, Rjwilmsi, Robert1947, Robh21, Rofl, RonFedericci, Ronz, Rosemaryamey, Runningmoose91, Samsknee, Sardanaphalus, Sarner, Schneelocke, Sean D Martin, Shawn in Montreal, Sirkad, Sketch, Sky Diva, Smalldumb, Some jerk on the Internet, Someguy1221, Spitfire, Sross (Public Policy), Steelpanther24, StephenBuxton, Storkynoob, Student7, Synapse001, Tabletop, Telsa, Tgrazio, The Nut, Tide rolls, Tittamiire, Tnxman307, Tobit2, Toetoetoetoe, Tombomp, Tommylommykins, Tonto35, Tony1379, Tpbradbury, Trusilver, Twinsday, Vampyrecat, Versageek, Viridian, Vorpalbla, Wasted Time R, Werdan7, Wes177, Whiskey in the Jar, WikHead, WikiJedits, Wo0dstock79, Wrelwser43, Yaroslav K, Yonidebest, YorkieDoctor, Zodon, 464 anonymous edits

Stepfamily *Source*: http://en.wikipedia.org/w/index.php?title=Stepfamily *Contributors*: 123william, 16@r, A little insignificant, Aaron Kauppi, Abby 94, Abd, Academic Challenger, Acather96, AndrewH, Antrophica, Aparna rajesh, April Is Really Fooled, Athanasius1, AussieBoy, BD2412, BDBWife, Barek, Ben Tibbetts, BigHaz, Binksternet, Blendedfamily, Blendedfamilyfun, BlueZenith, Bmf777, Bobblehead, Bobo192, Bogdangiusca, Bondedfamily, Booyabazooka, Branddobbe, Bssilverman, BuzyBody, CaroleHenson, CesarB, Chowbok, Clio the Muse, Closedmouth, Colonies Chris, Ddawson, DocWatson42, Doive, Ecuadoriangirl1986, Flammingo, Frecklefoot, Freedomworks, Gary2863, George Ho, Gogo Dodo, Golbez, Goldfritha, Gregoryjames, HistoryBA, Hu12, Ivysaur, JAF1970, JHunterJ, Jademw, Jattwarcraft, JeffJ, Jhenderson777, Jpbjoel, JzG, Kajasudhakarababu, Kalimac, Katieh5584, Katlr, Kelisi, LA2, Leininge, Lightmouse, Longhair, Loomis51, Lord Opeth, Lord of Night, MER-C, Man vyi, Marek69, Maxrandom777, MegX, Megland, MelanieN, MeltBanana, Michael A. White, Mipadi, Miquonranger03, Missdipsy, Moshe Constantine Hassan Al-Silverburg, Murmuration, Myles Callum, Namangwari, NawlinWiki, Nbarth, Neelix, Ngmpep, Nights Not End, Nominalthesecond, Novalis, Oda Mari, Owen, PaoloNapolitano, Patrick, Penbat, Phirazo, Pilgrim27, Psiphiorg, Psycho275, R'n'B, Redforza21, RepublicanJacobite, ReyBrujo, Richard001, Rixs, Rjwilmsi, RobertCMWV1974, Rossford, Rōnin, SL93, STEVE SURE, Sanser101, Sanspeur, Scchristianafvet, SchreiberBike, SchuminWeb, Secondwife, Serpent's Choice, Shalom Yechiel, ShelfSkewed, Shell Kinney, SimonP, Sirrion, Sjb64579, Sotakeit, Spanish lullaby, Stepadoptionblog, Stepfamily scotland, Steptopia, StuRat, Superstep, SusanGTD, TakuyaMurata, Tassedethe, The Squicks, Tijfo098, Timrollpickering, Triddle, Trivialist, USN1977, Uvahoo, ViperSnake151, Vkt183, Volcanictelephone, Vzbs34, Wikidestroyer44, Zachlipton, Zestos, Zuejay, Писатель А, 163 anonymous edits

Embryo_transfer *Source*: http://en.wikipedia.org/w/index.php?title=Embryo_transfer *Contributors*: 28421u2232nfenfcenc, ALEXEIS, ATaccount, Alberrosidus, Ankit Maity, Arcadian, Atulsnischal, Bpeps, Btxob, Cgoodwin, Chungalin, Crazy Boris with a red beard, Doniago, Ekem, Epolk, Eponimm, Ernie83, Favonian, FertilityPlan, George100, Gilliam, HFEA, Harayda, Howcheng, Htct56, Hu12, Hydrogen Iodide, Icarus3, JP ID MC, Jdavidb, Jfurr1981, Joe407, Lahiru k, Lesswealth, LilHelpa, Lindsaywells, MER-C, Mack2, Majikjeff, Mambocabo, Melaen, Michael Hardy, Mikael Häggström, Mike Rosoft, Mild Bill Hiccup, Mwanner, Nsaa, Ozkan199, PGWG, Pete.Hurd, PigFlu Oink, Piledhigheranddeeper, QuizzicalBee, R'n'B, Rami radwan, Rich Farmbrough, Richard Arthur Norton (1958-), Rjwilmsi, Saguair, Sam Hocevar, SasiSasi, Snalwibma, Spangineer, Spotfixer, Surrogatemom, Technostorks, Tellyaddict, Tins128, Tlesher, Tombomp, Tommy2010, Waffles19941618, WikiDao, Woohookitty, Xenobiologista, 97 anonymous edits

Egg_donation *Source*: http://en.wikipedia.org/w/index.php?title=Egg_donation *Contributors*: *Kat*, Alansohn, Andie-Portland, Anon16510, Anthonyhcole, Arcadian, Aviad2001, Baby2mom, Barek, Belovedfreak, Bloggeroo, Bobo192, Boghog, Btxob, CanadianLinuxUser, Charlieemurray, Christopheredwin, Coastdigital, Cosmic Latte, DBigXray, Daughter of Mímir, David Levy, Dgmoran, Drbenjaminsmith, Dzigunenko, Ekem, EnakoNosaj, Eperotao, Fightblognet, Fixiemama, Flavio Fernandez, Giraffedata, Hu12, Icarus3, Infertilityws, Infnetwk, IronGargoyle, JennKitten, Jess129, Jhanrahan, Jobxyz, Keilana, Kencf0618, Kjlewis, Krissf, L Kensington, Lindsayjones1995, Luckas Blade, Lzcrane, MAFeinman, Mandarax, Marnad1963, Mehrunes Dagon, Michaeldonor, Mikael Häggström, Ml66uk2, Novergrael, Pairadox, Photouploaded, Plasticspork, Puddleglum, Rachaelzi, Rachinbar, Richard001, Rjwilmsi, Saguair, SchreiberBike, Shaliya waya, Srose, StarDigian, Starinis, Subversive.sound, SuperHamster, Tcncv, Teesquire, Thayvian, The Gamma King, The Thing That Should Not Be, Tide rolls, Tmax64, Tobor0, Toni PC, Versageek, Vlanery, WhatamIdoing, Zandperl, 133 anonymous edits

List_of_Mendelian_traits_in_humans *Source*: http://en.wikipedia.org/w/index.php?title=List_of_Mendelian_traits_in_humans *Contributors*: Abductive, Adrigon, Aero13792468, Akshit Goyal, Alansohn, Amakuha, Arjayay, Asclepius, Bensin, Calgary, Cancun771, Fences and windows, Gawaxay, Glagolev, Grow60, Gwicky, HappyCamper, Iampied, Jcatgrl, Jfdwolff, Jnnfrdndr, Joyous!, Jwarhol, Lucid, Marek69, Matstuff, Pete.Hurd, Primalmoon, Qrthgrtd the Second, SMcCandlish, Scapler, Severa, Silvermen, Stevvers, Thumperward, YakbutterT, 74 anonymous edits

Earlobe *Source*: http://en.wikipedia.org/w/index.php?title=Earlobe *Contributors*: 10metreh, 5 albert square, 5Q5, Adam Bishop, Adambrowne666, Adamg4, Ahuds, Alansohn, Albajessica, Alivemajor, Alphathon, AnakngAraw, Animeronin, Animum, Arcadian, Astrometrics, Astroview120mm, AuburnPilot, Axeman89, Axl, Babbage, Beno1000, Bensin, Berean Hunter, CalumH93, Carlos is64, Childear, Cometstyles, Cool3, Courcelles, Cybergirl215, DMacks, DanielCD, DbelangeA, Dgw, DictionScholars, Discospinster, Dougiefresh27, Drunkchipmunk, Dstrek, ESkog, Earpol, Edderso, Eliz81, Emrayson, Erik Carson, Favonian, Fishal, Fre k, FreplySpang, Fruitgo1, Gimmetrow, Gogo Dodo, Hallows AG, HannaLi, Harry, Highway666, Hintha, Hjfreyer, Horse2954, Innes6087, Itsmeiam, J.delanoy, Jedravent, Jeff G., Jusdafax, Justsail, KTC, Kauczuk, Kazkaskazkasako, KnowledgeOfSelf, Kukini, Kuru, Legend tracker, Littlegirlearspierced, Loggie, Mangoe, Mavigogun, Maxn919, Mermaid from the Baltic Sea, Miranda, MuZemike, Much noise, NawlinWiki, Niceguyedc, Nick1nildram, Nicke L, Nina90, Nitishkorula, North Alabama 000, OwenX, Paul Davidson, Portillo, Professorsrini, Prolog, Qxz, R000t, RDBrown, Rich Farmbrough, Rklawton, Rm1271, Rolando, Rrburke, Rror, Rtivey01, Sam Korn, Sazaja, Sfahey, Sgosnipes, Sheogorath, Shoeofdeath, Skaffman, SkyWalker, Slightsmile, Tahmidal Zami, Taktoa, Tannim101, The sock that should not be, TheCamelKiller, Thw1309, Tide rolls, TomHaffie, Tumadoireacht, Umbriel, Vanished user 03, Victor, Vivaldi, W guice, West.andrew.g, Yomomz1, 187 anonymous edits

Image Sources, Licenses and Contributors

File:Under the horse chestnut tree2.jpg *Source*: http://en.wikipedia.org/w/index.php?title=File:Under_the_horse_chestnut_tree2.jpg *License*: unknown *Contributors*: Berrucomons, Durova, George Ho, Homonihilis, Julia W, Killiondude, Kilom691, Kozuch, Mattes, Miya

File:Maapay tay Kaka.jpg *Source*: http://en.wikipedia.org/w/index.php?title=File:Maapay_tay_Kaka.jpg *License*: unknown *Contributors*: User:Khalid Mahmood

File:wikisource-logo.svg *Source*: http://en.wikipedia.org/w/index.php?title=File:Wikisource-logo.svg *License*: unknown *Contributors*: Nicholas Moreau

File:Frog in frogspawn.jpg *Source*: http://en.wikipedia.org/w/index.php?title=File:Frog_in_frogspawn.jpg *License*: unknown *Contributors*: User:Salimfadhley

File:Lynch Armenia Five generations.png *Source*: http://en.wikipedia.org/w/index.php?title=File:Lynch_Armenia_Five_generations.png *License*: unknown *Contributors*: Harry Finnis Blosse Lynch

Image:Baby Mother Grandmother and Great Grandmother.jpg *Source*: http://en.wikipedia.org/w/index.php?title=File:Baby_Mother_Grandmother_and_Great_Grandmother.jpg *License*: unknown *Contributors*: User:Azoreg

File:MocheCeramicBirth.jpg *Source*: http://en.wikipedia.org/w/index.php?title=File:MocheCeramicBirth.jpg *License*: unknown *Contributors*: Pattych (talk). Original uploader was Pattych at en.wikipedia

Image:Eucharius Rößlin Rosgarten Childbirth.jpg *Source*: http://en.wikipedia.org/w/index.php?title=File:Eucharius_Rößlin_Rosgarten_Childbirth.jpg *License*: unknown *Contributors*: AndreasPraefcke, Bohème, FA2010, Testus, Thib Phil, הרטפואלק

Image:HumanNewborn.JPG *Source*: http://en.wikipedia.org/w/index.php?title=File:HumanNewborn.JPG *License*: unknown *Contributors*: Ernest F

Image:Postpartum baby3.jpg *Source*: http://en.wikipedia.org/w/index.php?title=File:Postpartum_baby3.jpg *License*: unknown *Contributors*: FlickreviewR, Melimama, Para, Schekinov Alexey Victorovich, הרטפואלק

File:Gene.png *Source*: http://en.wikipedia.org/w/index.php?title=File:Gene.png *License*: unknown *Contributors*: Courtesy: National Human Genome Research Institute

File:DNA chemical structure.svg *Source*: http://en.wikipedia.org/w/index.php?title=File:DNA_chemical_structure.svg *License*: unknown *Contributors*: Hystrix, Madprime, Wickey, 5 anonymous edits

File:Gene2-plain.svg *Source*: http://en.wikipedia.org/w/index.php?title=File:Gene2-plain.svg *License*: unknown *Contributors*: User:Forluvoft

File:Rna-codons-protein.png *Source*: http://en.wikipedia.org/w/index.php?title=File:Rna-codons-protein.png *License*: unknown *Contributors*: DBooth, Monkeybait, Opabinia regalis

Image:Gregor Mendel.png *Source*: http://en.wikipedia.org/w/index.php?title=File:Gregor_Mendel.png *License*: unknown *Contributors*: Common Good, Editor at Large, Kilom691, Liberal Freemason, QWerk, Savh, TimVickers, Wilfredor, 4 anonymous edits

File:Punnett square mendel flowers.svg *Source*: http://en.wikipedia.org/w/index.php?title=File:Punnett_square_mendel_flowers.svg *License*: unknown *Contributors*: User:Madprime

File:Human genome by functions.svg *Source*: http://en.wikipedia.org/w/index.php?title=File:Human_genome_by_functions.svg *License*: unknown *Contributors*: User:Mikael Häggström

File:Foster care length of stay.gif *Source*: http://en.wikipedia.org/w/index.php?title=File:Foster_care_length_of_stay.gif *License*: unknown *Contributors*: Adoption and Foster Care Analysis and Reporting System U.S. Government

File:Childrens migrant programme.jpg *Source*: http://en.wikipedia.org/w/index.php?title=File:Childrens_migrant_programme.jpg *License*: unknown *Contributors*: 7mike5000, Fastilysock

Image:PTSD stress brain.gif *Source*: http://en.wikipedia.org/w/index.php?title=File:PTSD_stress_brain.gif *License*: unknown *Contributors*: National Institutes of Health

File:Riischildren.jpg *Source*: http://en.wikipedia.org/w/index.php?title=File:Riischildren.jpg *License*: unknown *Contributors*: Jacob Riis (May 3, 1849 - May 26, 1914)

File:Terrell Peterson.jpg *Source*: http://en.wikipedia.org/w/index.php?title=File:Terrell_Peterson.jpg *License*: unknown *Contributors*: 7mike5000, Melesse, Salavat

File:Yesoda-krishna.jpg *Source*: http://en.wikipedia.org/w/index.php?title=File:Yesoda-krishna.jpg *License*: unknown *Contributors*: Redtigerxyz, Roland zh, Sridhar1000

Image:Franz Jüttner Schneewittchen 8.jpg *Source*: http://en.wikipedia.org/w/index.php?title=File:Franz_Jüttner_Schneewittchen_8.jpg *License*: unknown *Contributors*: AndreasPraefcke, Mutter Erde

Image:Awake Groa Awake Mother - John Bauer.jpg *Source*: http://en.wikipedia.org/w/index.php?title=File:Awake_Groa_Awake_Mother_-_John_Bauer.jpg *License*: unknown *Contributors*: Aavindraa, Bloodofox, Goldfritha, Holt, Lokal Profil, Skipjack, Wst

File:Embryo, 8 cells.jpg *Source*: http://en.wikipedia.org/w/index.php?title=File:Embryo,_8_cells.jpg *License*: unknown *Contributors*: User:ekem

File:Embryo transfered calves.JPG *Source*: http://en.wikipedia.org/w/index.php?title=File:Embryo_transfered_calves.JPG *License*: unknown *Contributors*: User:Cgoodwin

Image:Hitchhiker's thumbs.jpg *Source*: http://en.wikipedia.org/w/index.php?title=File:Hitchhiker's_thumbs.jpg *License*: unknown *Contributors*: Adrigon

Image:Gray904.png *Source*: http://en.wikipedia.org/w/index.php?title=File:Gray904.png *License*: unknown *Contributors*: Arcadian, Iainf, Jacklee, M.Komorniczak, Mattes, Mike.lifeguard

Image:Earlobefreephoto.jpg *Source*: http://en.wikipedia.org/w/index.php?title=File:Earlobefreephoto.jpg *License*: unknown *Contributors*: Hjfreyer

Image:TattooedAttachedEarlobe.png *Source*: http://en.wikipedia.org/w/index.php?title=File:TattooedAttachedEarlobe.png *License*: unknown *Contributors*: Hjfreyer

Image:Tutankhamun Mask.JPG *Source*: http://en.wikipedia.org/w/index.php?title=File:Tutankhamun_Mask.JPG *License*: unknown *Contributors*: G.dallorto, Neithsabes, Nicor, Yippie, 1 anonymous edits

MIX
Papier aus verantwortungsvollen Quellen
Paper from responsible sources
FSC® C105338

Printed by Books on Demand GmbH, Norderstedt / Germany